Clinical Neurology

Guest Editors

THOMAS J. DIVERS, DVM
AMY L. JOHNSON, DVM

VETERINARY CLINICS OF NORTH AMERICA: EQUINE PRACTICE

www.vetequine.theclinics.com

Consulting Editor
ANTHONY SIMON TURNER, BVSc, MS

December 2011 • Volume 27 • Number 3

SAUNDERS an imprint of ELSEVIER, Inc.

W.B. SAUNDERS COMPANY
A Division of Elsevier Inc.

1600 John F. Kennedy Boulevard • Suite 1800 • Philadelphia, Pennsylvania 19103

http://www.vetequine.theclinics.com

VETERINARY CLINICS OF NORTH AMERICA: EQUINE PRACTICE Volume 27, Number 3
December 2011 ISSN 0749-0739, ISBN-13: 978-1-4557-7996-3

Editor: John Vassallo; j.vassallo@elsevier.com
Developmental Editor: Donald Mumford

Veterinary Clinics of North America: Equine Practice (ISSN 0749-0739) is published in April, August, and December by Elsevier Inc., 360 Park Avenue South, New York, NY 10010-1710. Business and Editorial Offices: 1600 John F. Kennedy Blvd., Suite 1800, Philadelphia, PA 19103-2899. Subscription prices are $257.00 per year (domestic individuals), $397.00 per year (domestic institutions), $126.00 per year (domestic students/residents), $299.00 per year (Canadian individuals), $496.00 per year (Canadian institutions), $346.00 per year (international individuals), $496.00 per year (international institutions), and $172.00 per year (international and Canadian students/residents). To receive student/resident rate, orders must be accompanied by name of affiliated institution, date of term, and the signature of program/residency coordinator on institution letterhead. Orders will be billed at individual rate until proof of status is received. Foreign air speed delivery is included in all *Clinics* subscription prices. All prices are subject to change without notice. **POSTMASTER:** Send address changes to *Veterinary Clinics of North America: Equine Practice*, 3251 Riverport Lane, Maryland Heights, MO 63043. Customer Service (orders, claims, online, change of address): Elsevier Health Sciences Division, Subscription Customer Service, 3251 Riverport Lane, Maryland Heights, MO 63043. Tel: 1-800-654-2452 (U.S. and Canada); 314-447-8871 (outside U.S. and Canada). Fax: 314-447-8029. E-mail: journalscustomerservice-usa@elsevier.com (for print support); E-mail: journalsonlinesupport-usa@elsevier (for online support).

Reprints. For copies of 100 or more of articles in this publication, please contact the Commercial Reprints Department, Elsevier Inc., 360 Park Avenue South, New York, NY 10010-1710. Tel.: 212-633-3812; Fax: 212-462-1935; E-mail: reprints@elsevier.com.

Veterinary Clinics of North America: Equine Practice is covered in *MEDLINE/PubMed (Index Medicus), Excerpta Medica, Current Contents/Agriculture, Biology and Environmental Sciences, and ISI.*

Printed and bound by CPI Group (UK) Ltd, Croydon, CR0 4YY

Transferred to Digital Print 2011

Contributors

CONSULTING EDITOR

ANTHONY SIMON TURNER, BVSc, MS
Diplomate, American College of Veterinary Surgeons; Professor, Department of Clinical Sciences, College of Veterinary Medicine and Biomedical Sciences, Colorado State University, Fort Collins, Colorado

GUEST EDITORS

THOMAS J. DIVERS, DVM
Diplomate, American College of Veterinary Internal Medicine; Diplomate, American College of Veterinary Emergency and Critical Care; Professor of Medicine, Department of Clinical Sciences, College of Veterinary Medicine, Cornell University, Ithaca, New York

AMY L. JOHNSON, DVM
Diplomate of American College of Veterinary Internal Medicine (Large Animal Internal Medicine); Assistant Professor of Large Animal Neurology and Medicine, Department of Clinical Studies - New Bolton Center, University of Pennsylvania School of Veterinary Medicine, Kennett Square, Pennsylvania

AUTHORS

MONICA ALEMAN, MVZ, PhD
Diplomate, American College of Veterinary Internal Medicine (Large Animal Internal Medicine); Neurology and Neurosurgery Resident III, Laboratories of Clinical Neurophysiology and Neuromuscular Disease, William R. Pritchard Veterinary Medical Teaching Hospital, School of Veterinary Medicine, University of California, Davis, California

ALEXANDRE S. BORGES, DVM, MS, PhD
Professor of Large Animal Internal Medicine, Department of Veterinary Clinical Science, College of Veterinary Medicine and Animal Science, São Paulo State University, Botucatu-SP, Brazil

DOMINIC R. DAWSON, DVM
Diplomate, American College of Veterinary Internal Medicine; Associate Veterinarian, Department of Medicine and Epidemiology, William R. Pritchard Veterinary Medical Teaching Hospital, School of Veterinary Medicine, University of California, Davis, California

THOMAS J. DIVERS, DVM
Diplomate, American College of Veterinary Internal Medicine; Diplomate, American College of Veterinary Emergency and Critical Care; Professor of Medicine, Department of Clinical Sciences, College of Veterinary Medicine, Cornell University, Ithaca, New York

SUE J. DYSON, MA, VetMB, PhD, FRCVS
Head of Clinical Orthopaedics, Centre for Equine Studies, Animal Health Trust, Lanwades Park, Kentford, Newmarket, Suffolk, England

Contributors

RACHEL B. GARDNER, DVM
Diplomate, American College of Veterinary Internal Medicine; B.W. Furlong &
Associates, Oldwick, New Jersey

NITA L. IRBY, DVM
Diplomate, American College of Veterinary Ophthalmologists; Lecturer, Department of
Clinical Sciences, College of Veterinary Medicine, Cornell University, Ithaca, New York

AMY L. JOHNSON, DVM
Diplomate of American College of Veterinary Internal Medicine (Large Animal Internal
Medicine); Assistant Professor of Large Animal Neurology and Medicine, Department of
Clinical Studies - New Bolton Center, University of Pennsylvania School of Veterinary
Medicine, Kennett Square, Pennsylvania

THERESIA F. LICKA, Dr med vet, Mag med vet, MRCVS
Clinic for Orthopedics in Ungulates, Department for Small Animals and Horses, University
of Veterinary Medicine, Vienna, Vienna, Austria; Honorary Fellow at the Royal (Dick)
School of Veterinary Studies, University of Edinburgh, Scotland, United Kingdom

PETER V. SCRIVANI, DVM,
Diplomate, American College of Veterinary Radiology; Assistant Professor of Veterinary
Imaging, Department of Clinical Sciences, College of Veterinary Medicine, Cornell
University, Ithaca, New York

MARCOS J. WATANABE, DVM, MS, PhD
Professor of Large Animal Surgery, Departments of Veterinary Surgery and
Anesthesiology, College of Veterinary Medicine and Animal Science, São Paulo State
University, Botucatu-SP, Brazil

Contents

Normal gait pattern and posture depend on an intact musculoskeletal and neural system, and deficits in either can lead to abnormal movements. The discrimination between neurologic and orthopedic causes can be difficult, and this text aims at describing some practical aspects and tests, which may be helpful for further differentiation. Not many studies have tried to identify measurable differences between neurologically normal, lame, and ataxic horses, and with the wider distribution of movement analysis systems, such studies will hopefully be carried out in due course.

Lesions of the neck are an uncommon primary cause of pain resulting in either lameness or poor performance but should be considered if local analgesic techniques of the limbs fail to abolish lameness or if there are clinical signs directly referable to the neck such as pain, abnormal neck posture, stiffness, or patchy sweating.

Modern neuroimaging technologies produce exquisite images of patient morphology and function, as well as store and distribute information more efficiently. Advanced equine neuroimaging is a specialized field that has unique challenges but provides a lot of useful information that is important for making a diagnosis, planning treatment, or providing prognostic information to guide owner choices regarding patient care. Optimizing equine neuroimaging starts with selecting an appropriate examination, understanding the capabilities of the different technologies, understanding normal anatomy and pathogenesis, and having a systematic approach to reviewing the images.

A complete neuro-ophthalmologic assessment is relatively simple, requires minimal instrumentation and should be performed as part of every complete ophthalmic and neurologic examination. This article summarizes the elements of the complete neuro-ophthalmologic examination of the equine patient, discusses selected causes of sudden blindness in the horse and discusses some common neuro-ophthalmic conditions, such as facial nerve paralysis, that have significant ophthalmic consequences.

The neuromuscular system is an important component of the nervous system. This system is composed of motor units. A motor unit consists of a single lower motor neuron, its axon and supportive cells (Schwann cells), neuromuscular junction, and all the muscle fibers innervated by the motor neuron. Signs of dysfunction can vary depending on the specific area affected. Lower motor neuron dysfunction results in muscle weakness, paresis to paralysis, decreased muscle tone, decreased to absent reflexes, and neurogenic muscle atrophy. This article reviews the neuromuscular region and function, dysfunction, clinical signs associated with specific disorders, and diagnostic workup.

This article provides an overview of the more common toxins and adverse drug reactions, along with more rare toxins and reactions that result in neurologic dysfunction in horses. A wide variety of symptoms, treatments, and outcomes are seen with toxic neurologic disease in horses. An in-depth history and thorough physical examination are needed to determine if a toxin or an adverse drug reaction is responsible for the clinical signs. Once a toxin or adverse drug reaction is identified, the specific antidote, if available, and supportive care should be administered promptly.

Examination, management and treatment of recumbent horses have become more common in recent years. As nutrition and management practices improve and the life span of horses increases, recumbency due to age-related disorders has become more common. The increasingly growing perception of horses as companion animals has also resulted in a larger proportion of horses that are evaluated and treated for recumbency, regardless of the economic value of the animal.

Assessment and management of recumbent horses are challenging, and potentially expensive and dangerous. Equine veterinarians must have the skills to properly evaluate, manage, and facilitate transport of these patients.

Several diseases of the guttural pouches have been described in the literature, and the comprehensive evaluation of these structures is an important element of the clinical exam. Guttural pouch abnormalities form part of an important group of differential diagnoses for horses presenting dysphagia, cough, fever, nasal discharge, epistaxis, and abnormal cranial nerve function. This text will address the descriptive anatomy of the guttural pouch, emphasizing the nervous structures in direct contact with it and the possible neurologic signs resulting from disease. We will also review the major literature regarding guttural pouch diseases associated with neurologic abnormalities.

The equine nervous system may be infected by several different types of organisms, including viruses, bacteria, protozoa, nematodes, and fungi. One of the fundamental principles of neurology is that clinical signs reflect the location of the lesion rather than the etiology. Therefore, elucidating the cause of disease necessitates specific ante-mortem (and sometimes post-mortem) diagnostic testing. This article reviews the most common agents that affect the equine nervous system in North America, focusing on recent advances in diagnosis and treatment.

Metabolic encephalopathy can be defined as cerebral dysfunction that occurs in response to endogenously derived biochemical abnormalities. There are only a small number of metabolic disorders known to cause clinically relevant encephalopathy in horses. Resulting clinical signs are often dramatic and may include blindness, bizarre behavior, seizures, depression, and coma. The most common metabolic disorders causing encephalopathy in horses are: primary hyperammonemia syndromes, hepatoencephalopathy, uremic encephalopathy, sodium and glucose concentration abnormalities, neonatal encephalopathy, kernicterus, and hypocalcemic seizures.

FORTHCOMING ISSUES

April 2012

Therapeutic Farriery
Stephen E. O'Grady, DVM, MRCVS, and
Andrew Parks, VetMB, MS, MRCVS,
Guest Editors

August 2012

Equine Ambulatory Practice
David Ramey, DVM, and
Mark R. Baus, DVM, *Guest Editors*

December 2012

Advances in Equine Imaging
Natasha Werpy, DVM, and
Myra Barrett, DVM, MS, *Guest Editors*

RECENT ISSUES

August 2011

Cell-based Therapies in Orthopedics
Matthew C. Stewart, BVSc,
MVetClinStud, PhD, and
Allison A. Stewart, DVM, MS,
Guest Editors

April 2011

Endocrine Diseases
Ramiro E. Toribio, DVM, MS, PhD,
Guest Editor

December 2010

**Pain in Horses: Physiology Pathophysiology
and Therapeutic Implications**
William W. Muir, DVM, PhD, *Guest Editor*

RELATED INTEREST

Veterinary Clinics of North America: Small Animal Practice
September 2010 (Vol. 40, No. 5)
Spinal Diseases
Ronaldo C. da Costa, DMV, MSc, PhD, *Guest Editor*

THE CLINICS ARE NOW AVAILABLE ONLINE!

Access your subscription at:
www.theclinics.com

Preface

Clinical Neurology

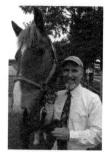 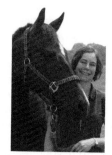

Thomas J. Divers, DVM   Amy L. Johnson, DVM
Guest Editors

Equine neurology is one of the most fascinating and challenging aspects of equine practice. Neurologic disorders can affect any age horse and can result from many different infectious and noninfectious causes. The horse's nervous system extends throughout the body and, when diseased, may cause a variety of clinical signs depending on which segments of the nervous system are involved. Even after a thorough neurologic examination, we may not be able to arrive at a specific diagnosis since clinical signs are sometimes subtle and often nonspecific for any one particular neurologic disease. There may be difficulty in determining if a gait abnormality is due to a neurologic or a musculoskeletal disease in some cases, and many neuroimaging techniques are not readily available to the practitioner. Progress is being made though, as recent advances in imaging, electromyelography, specific disease testing, and programmed gait analysis are improving our ability to diagnose neurologic dysfunction in the horse and determine specific causes. Additionally, we now better understand how important normal neck movement is to the horse's gait and that musculoskeletal diseases of the neck may cause gait abnormalities that can often be confused with spinal cord disease.

Two of the most controversial and written-about disorders in the horse, equine protozoal myeloencephalitis and equine herpesvirus 1, are both infectious neurologic disorders with frequent new discoveries being made from ongoing research. Rabies, another infectious disease of the nervous system, will always be of special concern to the equine practitioner due to its zoonotic potential. Encephalopathic diseases and blindness caused by neurologic disorders in the horse often have acute and dramatic clinical signs, sometimes making it difficult to safely approach and treat those horses. Bizarre behavior and other neurologic signs due to cerebral or neuromuscular dysfunction may also occur as a result of adverse drug reactions or intoxication. Another very interesting and species-unique aspect of equine neurology is that

Vet Clin Equine 27 (2011) ix–x
doi:10.1016/j.cveq.2011.08.011
0749-0739/11/$ – see front matter © 2011 Elsevier Inc. All rights reserved.

vetequine.theclinics.com

peripheral neuropathies may occur secondary to guttural pouch disorders and temporohyoid arthropathy.

It is not possible in this issue to cover all diseases of the equine nervous system. Instead, our goal here is to provide information on various aspects of the equine nervous system that may not be commonly covered in-depth in textbooks or conferences and to provide updates on other frequently discussed disorders. We would like to thank all the wonderful authors who have taken time out of their busy schedules to write articles and share their knowledge.

We hope you will find these articles useful in your practice and to be of help in diagnosing and treating neurologic conditions in the horse. We would like to thank all those veterinarians interested in neurology who have previously contributed information on the equine nervous system in textbooks, scientific publications, and conference presentations. We are hesitant to name those many individuals who have contributed so much to our understanding of neurology for fear of leaving someone out and you already know from your readings of their articles and textbooks and attending conferences who these individuals are. We would, though, like to recognize Dr Alexander de Lahunta and Dr Jill Beech, who helped pioneer the field of equine neurology and had a big influence on both of our careers. Thank you "Dr D" and Dr Beech and to all fellow equine practitioners; happy reading about the following selected aspects of equine neurology.

Thomas J. Divers, DVM
Department of Clinical Sciences
College of Veterinary Medicine
Cornell University
Ithaca, NY 14853, USA

Amy L. Johnson, DVM
Department of Clinical Studies - New Bolton Center
University of Pennsylvania School of Veterinary Medicine
382 West Street Road
Kennett Square, PA 19348, USA

E-mail addresses:
tjd8@cornell.edu (T.J. Divers)
amyjohn@vet.upenn.edu (A.L. Johnson)

Differentiation of Ataxic and Orthopedic Gait Abnormalities in the Horse

Theresia F. Licka, Dr med vet, Mag med vet, MRCVS[a,b]

KEYWORDS

- Equine lameness • Equine ataxia • Neurology
- Orthopedics • Wobbler

Movement and, to some degree, posture at stance or even in recumbency depends on the functionality, interaction, and integration of the passive and active musculo-skeletal structures, with pattern generation, motor innervation, and proprioception as the relevant neurologic aspects. Any abnormality within this arrangement will lead to a gait or movement deficit, and complex interactions can be present, such as the reduction of proprioceptive input due to damage of sensory nerves associated with orthopedic disease. A possible explanation for the slapping hoof placement in horses with laminitis, which was described to be similar to the gait of some "wobblers,"[1] could therefore be the damage to the sensory nerve fibers associated with pedal bone displacement and laminar disruption. An additional complicating factor is the increased incidence of orthopedic trauma and/or disease in neurologically impaired horses, as they are more prone to falling, stumbling, slipping, etc, than neurologically intact horses. In such cases, a degree of orthopedic pain may accompany ataxia.

STANCE

While the postural sway in healthy young horses was described to be very consistent,[2] this has not yet been measured in ataxic or lame horses, and the following information on horses is therefore based on clinical experience. *At stance, most orthopedic, pain-related disorders will produce a uniform, consistent posture, which reduces discomfort during standing.* If more than one limb is affected, weight-shifting and alternating resting of limbs may occur. If the horse is turned or backed, a similar body position will be reached. *This is different from ataxia, where the center of gravity of the body is not supported consistently with the same limb arrangement, but with a larger variety of limb positions.* After any intervention, such as a tail-pull or a gentle

---

The author has nothing to disclose.

[a] Department for Small Animals and Horses, Orthopedics in Ungulates, Equine Surgery, Veterinaerplatz 1, Veterinary University Vienna, Vienna A-1210, Austria
[b] Royal (Dick) School of Veterinary Studies, University of Edinburgh, Scotland, UK
E-mail address: theresia.licka@vetmeduni.ac.at

rocking of the pelvis, the resulting limb positions in relation to the trunk and limb orientations in relation to the body axis can be different from the original situation.

In lactating sows, the high correlation between abnormal posture and foot lesions has been documented, even though the type of abnormal posture was rather vaguely defined as "weight persistently unequally distributed, no weight borne on the affected limb or limb elevated from the ground.[3]" In cattle, the postural abnormality of arching the back was described as a rapid screening method for lameness.[4] In goats with transmissible spongiform encephalopathies, postural deficits described as a hunched appearance, with crouching or standing with the legs wide-based, were not found to be significantly more frequent than in control animals,[5] also indicating that these are transient phenomena in neurologic impairment. Also, such postural anomalies may have a low sensitivity for detection of encephalopathies.

Wide-based stance, especially of the hindlimbs, is commonly described in ataxic horses. This wide-based stance will increase the stability of stance, as the area of support under the center of gravity is increased, and it is probably the result of some residual sensation or awareness of being at risk of falling over. Only rarely will an orthopedic disorder produce a similar stance, if loading of the lateral aspects of the limbs is painful.

Practical Tests

Repeated, abrupt stops after turning or backing will accentuate variation in limb position, mainly hindlimb stance. A typical ataxic horse may end up with forelimbs and hindlimbs facing in up to 90°-different directions. Especially a variation in the loading pattern should be noted at stance, such as by evaluating the prominence of the extensor branches of the suspensory apparatus in the limbs. Also, the hindlimbs can be gently turned out by pushing the point of the hock toward medial. Crossing of the limbs is often possible in ataxic horses, but it may also be possible in pain-free cooperative horses. In a lame horse, this correction of limb position will often be carried out immediately, if it causes discomfort. In a neurologically intact horse, all abnormal limb positions will be corrected at the latest when another change of the body centre of gravity is triggered by, for example, clapping the hands and making the horse turn its head to listen or to follow a carrot.

MOTION

At slow speeds or in stance, neurologic abnormalities of movement are more commonly observed than at faster speeds. At walk on a treadmill, fuzzy clustering of kinematics of normal and ataxic horses using a simple set of body and limb markers was successfully used to differentiate the 2 groups.[6] Also, during walking on a treadmill, all intraindividual correlations between motion cycles of a single limb as well as between the 4 limbs were significantly different in ataxic horses, whereas at trot this was not detected in all correlations.[7] In investigating horses trotting over a force plate, the lateral force peak and the variation in vertical force peaks in both hindlimbs were significantly larger in ataxic horses than in neurologically intact sound or lame horses. In the lame horses, the vertical force was lower in the lame hindlimb.[8]

In all quadrupedal animals, moving at higher speeds depends largely on central pattern generation in the spinal cord. In the decerebrated cat, this central pattern generation for the hindlimbs has been localized to the lumbar spine using epidural stimulation in the cat[9] (ie, caudal to the typical site of spinal cord lesions in the horse). Central pattern generation is responsible for both the coordination of movement within a limb and the coordination of gait patterns between limbs. In health, the final motor output is shaped both by the central pattern generation and by the sensory feedback from peripheral receptors and reconfigured by neuromodulators,[10] which may be reduced or missing in neurologically impaired horses. Also, supraspinal inputs are essential for initiation of locomotion prior to central pattern generation as well as for the cessation of movement, and therefore at the beginning of movement or at a transition between gaits, ataxia can be noted more readily.

In a study investigating motor bias in ridden and unridden horses when challenged at canter on the lunge,[11] the times spent in canter, selecting the correct lead, and becoming disunited were documented. All of these characteristics have been described as indicators of balance in the horse,[12–14] and they were correlated with each other, without signs of left or right bias in either group of horses being documented. However, unridden horses were disunited more often than the ridden horses, showing their lack of coordination training in this difficult task. This is similar in ataxic horses, where the difficulty of cantering may also produce disunited canter, and disunited canter and correct canter will be seen in turn, as the consistent use of disunited canter also requires a degree of balance. On the contrary, horses with a single limb lameness will usually show persistent disunited canter when the horse is cantering on the ipsilateral rein. Additionally episodes of bunny hopping, that is (nearly) level placement of the hindlimbs at canter, will be more persistent in hindlimb lame horses than in ataxic horses. Challenging the horse on an incline at the walk will accentuate a hindlimb lameness uphill, and a forelimb lameness downhill due to the change in body mass carried by hind or forelimbs, but the effect of ataxia is less predictable.

Practical Tests

For differentiation between ataxic and lame horses, a slow walk including zigzagging and a number of walk trot transitions is advisable. Toe dragging is common in hindlimb lameness and may mimic hypometria. It is rare in forelimb lameness. Hypermetria of forelimbs or hindlimbs is mostly associated with neurologic abnormalities. At the beginning of walk and trot, a very different length of the first left and right stride may be noticed, as well as abnormal head and neck movement, indicating that momentum has to be gained in the front half of the horse. Similarly, at the end of trot, different stride lengths may be noted, and knuckling, as well as abrupt movements, may be present. Stumbling and slipping are also often obvious at the transitions. During trot, neurologic abnormalities may not be clear, but most weight-bearing lameness will become more prominent at trot due to the markedly increased forces transmitted via painful structures. Comparing the width of the hoof prints during a straight line of trot in hand by trotting over a freshly prepared soft surface may also be helpful. In a lame horse, often a single limb, usually the (most) affected one is placed farther away from the center of gravity of the body; in an ataxic horse, this will not be uniform over several strides. Also, on semisolid surfaces such as loamy ground or wet pressed sand, the variation in the depth of hoof prints at even trotting speed may also be varying from stride to stride, indicating ataxia. This is different from horses with a stabbing sudden onset of orthopedic pain, such as a mobile joint chip that gets caught in the sensitive area between bone and the joint capsule. After such a sudden onset, the horse takes at least several strides, often many minutes, to return to its original pattern of consistent asymmetric movement. At canter, again the trot–canter transitions are interesting, with persistent bunny hopping or reduced cranial placement of the inner hindlimb indicating lameness, whereas occasional changing between disunited canter and correct canter can be present in unschooled, normal, or ataxic horses. If the questionable ataxia and the surface used make the risk acceptable, cantering the horse on the lunge with full tension on the lunge that is suddenly released may also show a lack of coordination with sideway stumbling in ataxic horses. If horses are walked on an incline, repeated stops and turns should be carried out to further challenge its coordinative capacity.

EXERCISE

Most orthopedic diseases and disorders show a consistent relationship with exercise, with, for example, osteoarthritis typically improving with warming up or lameness associated with acute arthritis increasing during exercise. To assess whether such a repeatable relationship with exercise exists, several days of examination are ideal; alternatively, anamnestic information can be obtained from the trainer or rider of the horse. Riding a potentially ataxic horse is a grave risk for the rider and should not be part of the exercise investigation. In general, lame horses are more commonly reluctant to work or to continue to work than ataxic horses, where a disconcerting willingness to move can be associated with quite noticeable movement irregularities. In both groups of horses, exhaustion will occur prematurely, as the efficiency of locomotion is reduced both by ataxia (and possibly further impaired if ataxia is associated with weakness) due to the large variation of stride cycles and by lameness where the inadequate distribution of the work load onto the limbs leads to overexertion. Additionally, heart rate was documented to be elevated with lameness before, during, and after exercise in field training of racehorses.[15] If at all possible, it is advisable to avoid muscular fatigue and subsequent muscle pain, as this makes further investigations into the differentiation of orthopedic and neurologic problems more difficult, because the resulting stiffness and pain will blunt the differences. Resting the horse for 30 to 60 minutes after some exercise will change the gait pattern, yet again, in many orthopedic diseases and disorders, either increasing the lameness, especially when rested at stance in a cold environment, or improving the lameness, especially when rested at a gentle walk in a warm environment. Such effects are not commonly noted in ataxic horses.

SHORT-TERM MEDICATIONS

If pain-associated lameness is present, this can obviously be influenced by adequate pain relief. The most commonly used test for the differentiation between lameness and ataxia is therefore perineural and/or intrasynovial anesthesia, especially if it is carried out in more than one limb; for example, in cases of laminitis, questionable neurologic symptoms such as abnormal stance or increased impact on landing can be completely abolished. This proves the type of gait disorder to owner and examining veterinarian. However, many cases of lameness are partly mechanical (eg, due to a reduced range of motion of an osteoarthritic joint), and this aspect will not change with pain relief. Especially hindlimb lameness can often not be abolished with pain relief, probably due to the marked changes in the use of the muscles of the trunk and of both hindlimbs,[16] which even after a medium-term duration of lameness of 6 weeks does not allow return to perfectly normal locomotion without a short period of retraining.

In a model of short-term foot lameness, a single intravenous dose of phenylbutazone or flunixin meglumine was efficacious in reducing heart rate as well as clinical lameness score within 60 minutes.[17] Unfortunately, the lameness reduction is sometimes not as obvious in the typical clinical patient with chronic multilimb lameness; in these cases, an increased willingness to work is a more consistently seen immediate improvement with Nonsteroidal anti-inflammatory drugs (NSAIDs). No such change is usually noted in the pain-free ataxic horse. The later addition of strong analgesics such as opioids should be considered if the gait abnormality does not change with NSAID treatment. However, the possible slight changes in attitude such as euphoria and locomotor stimulation, as well as excitatory effects,[18] have to be taken into consideration, which may make a change in gait difficult to evaluate. Also, after opioids, repeat heart rate measurements may no longer be representative of the change in locomotory pain. Sedation with low doses of alpha- agonists has been shown not to change measured forelimb lameness parameters in horses trotting on a treadmill,[19] and the clinical evaluation of lameness may well be improved with mild sedation, especially in excited horses, due to the more consistent gait as the influence of external stimuli is reduced. In normal horses, sedation produces a gait abnormality roughly similar to ataxia,[7] and therefore ataxia may be increased in ataxic horses after sedation. If light sedation without the addition of opioids is carried out to, for example, obtain radiographs of the cervical spine,[20] the aftereffects of this should be used to reassess the horse at walk and trot, to allow a possibly increased lameness to become noted.

ADVANCED DIAGNOSTIC TESTS

In referral institutions, further workup may be carried out, which can include electromyography (EMG) of skeletal muscles, to differentiate between disuse atrophy and neurogenic atrophy. This has been successfully used in horses with suspected grass sickness, where EMG results were consistent with muscle biopsy findings of slight neurogenic atrophy.[21] Myotonic EMG discharges were also found to be present in cases of equine myotonic dystrophy, confirmed by histologic changes in skeletal muscles.[22] These results are promising; however, such tests have not been carried out in mild cervical ataxia, where differentiation between lameness and ataxia is most commonly needed, and where both cases show abnormalities in EMG characteristics of skeletal muscle.

Additionally, in select clinical settings, transcranial magnetic stimulation may be carried out to evaluate the integrity of spinal pathways. This has been successfully used in horses with cervical ataxia, which showed significantly different evoked motor responses compared to normal horses.[23]

SUMMARY

The differentiation of ataxia and orthopedic disease can be facilitated by the use of several additional tests, not commonly part of either neurologic or orthopedic examination protocols. However, a full neurologic and orthopedic examination and suitable diagnostic imaging will of course also be necessary in such cases. The common association of orthopedic and neurologic disease makes it even more necessary to correctly attribute movement or posture abnormalities to potentially treatable structures.

REFERENCES

1. Cripps PJ, Eustace RA. Factors involved in the prognosis of equine laminitis in the UK. Equ Vet J 1999;31(5):433–42.
2. Clayton HM, Bialski DE, Lanovaz JL, et al. Assessment of the reliability of a technique to measure postural sway in horses. Am J Vet Res 2003;64(11):1354–9.
3. Kilbride AL, Gillman CE, Green LE. A cross-sectional study of prevalence and risk factors for foot lesions and abnormal posture in lactating sows on commercial farms in England. Anim Welfare 2010;19(4):473–80.
4. Thomsen PT. Rapid screening method for lameness in dairy cows. Vet Rec 2009; 164(22):689–90.

5. Konold T, Bone GE, Phelan LJ, et al. Monitoring of clinical signs in goats with transmissible spongiform encephalopathies. BMC Vet Res 2010;6:13.

6. Keegan KG, Arafat S, Skubic M, et al. Detection of spinal ataxia in horses using fuzzy clustering of body position uncertainty. Equine Vet J 2004;36(8):712–7.

7. Strobach A, Kotschwar A, Mayhew IG, et al. Gait pattern of the ataxic horse compared to sedated and nonsedated horses. Equine Vet J 2006;(Suppl 36):423–6.

8. Ishihara A, Reed SM, Rajala-Schultz PJ, et al. Use of kinetic gait analysis for detection, quantification, and differentiation of hind limb lameness and spinal ataxia in horses. J Am Vet Med Assoc 2009;234(5):644–51.

9. Iwahara T, Atsuta Y, Garcia-Rill E, et al. Spinal cord stimulation-induced locomotion in the adult cat. Brain Res Bull 1992;28(1):99–105.

10. MacKay-Lyons M. Central pattern generation of locomotion: a review of the evidence. Phys Ther 2002;82(1):69–83.

11. Wells AED, Blache D. Horses do not exhibit motor bias when their balance is challenged. Animal Science 2008;2(11):1645–50.

12. Rees L. The fundamentals of riding. London: Roxby Paintbox Company; 1991.

13. Davis C. The kingdom of the horse. Sydney: New Holland Publishers Australia Pty Ltd; 1998.

14. Moffett H. Enlightened equitation. London: David and Charles; 1999.

15. Foreman JH, Bayly WM, Grant BD, et al. Standardized exercise test and daily heart rate responses of thoroughbreds undergoing conventional race training and detraining. Am J Vet Res 1990;51(6):914–20.

16. Zaneb H, Kaufmann V, Stanek C, et al. Quantitative differences in activities of back and pelvic limb muscles during walking and trotting between chronically lame and nonlame horses. Am J Vet Res 2009;70(9):1129–34.

17. Foreman JH, Grubb TL, Inoue OJ, et al. Efficacy of single-dose intravenous phenylbutazone and flunixin meglumine before, during and after exercise in an experimental reversible model of foot lameness in horses. Equine Vet J 2010;42(Suppl 38):601–5.

18. Clutton RE. Opioid analgesia in horses. Vet Clin North Am Equine Pract 2010;26(3):493–514.

19. Buchner HH, Kübber P, Zohmann E, et al. Sedation and antisedation as tools in equine lameness examination. Equine Vet J 1999;(Suppl 30):227–30.

20. Van Biervliet J. An evidence-based approach to clinical questions in the practice of equine neurology. Vet Clin North Am Equine Pract 2007;23(2):317–28.

21. Wijnberg ID, Franssen H, Jansen GH, et al. The role of quantitative electromyography (EMG) in horses suspected of acute and chronic grass sickness. Equine Vet J 2006;38(3):230–7.

22. Hegreberg GA, Reed SM. Skeletal muscle changes associated with equine myotonic dystrophy. Acta Neuropathol 1990;80(4):426–31.

23. Nollet H, Deprez P, Van Ham L, et al. The use of magnetic motor evoked potentials in horses with cervical spinal cord disease. Equine Vet J 2002;34(2):156–63.

Lesions of the Equine Neck Resulting in Lameness or Poor Performance

Sue J. Dyson, MA, VetMB, PhD, FRCVS

KEYWORDS

• Stiffness • Forelimb lameness • Cervical vertebrae • Ataxia

Lesions of the neck are uncommon causes of pain resulting in either lameness or poor performance.

FUNCTIONAL ANATOMY

The neck consists of 7 cervical vertebrae, which articulate by both intercentral articulations, and articular process joints (APJs) (sometimes called synovial intervertebral articulations) that have large joint capsules to accommodate the degree of movement between adjacent vertebrae. Interposed between the vertebral bodies are intervertebral fibrocartilages to which is attached the dorsal longitudinal ligament, which lies on the floor of the vertebral canal. The ligamentum flavum connects the arches of adjacent vertebrae. The atlas (the first cervical vertebra) and the axis (the second cervical vertebra) have a unique shape and specialized joints. The atlantooccipital joint is a ginglymus joint, which permits flexion and extension and also a small amount of lateral oblique movement. The atlantoaxial joint is a trochoid or pivot joint; the atlas and head rotate on the axis. The ligament of the dens is strong and fan shaped and extends from the dorsal surface of the odontoid peg (dens) to the ventral arch of the axis. The ligamentum nuchae extends from the occiput to the withers and consists of funicular and lamellar parts. The lamellar part separates the 2 lateral muscle groups. The atlantal bursa is interposed between the funicular part of the ligamentum nuchae and the dorsal arch of the atlas; a second bursa may exist between the ligament and the spine of the axis. The muscles of the neck can be divided into lateral and ventral groups. The neck has 8 cervical nerves, the first of which emerges through the lateral foramen of the atlas, the second between the atlas and the axis, and the eighth between the seventh cervical vertebra and the first thoracic vertebra. The sixth to eighth cervical nerves contribute to the brachial plexus.

The author has nothing to disclose.
Centre for Equine Studies, Animal Health Trust, Lanwades Park, Kentford, Newmarket, Suffolk, CB8 7UU, England
E-mail address: sue.dyson@aht.org.uk

Vet Clin Equine 27 (2011) 417–437
doi:10.1016/j.cveq.2011.08.005
0749-0739/11/$ – see front matter © 2011 Elsevier Inc. All rights reserved.

HISTORY AND CLINICAL SIGNS GIVING RISE TO A SUSPICION OF A NECK-RELATED PROBLEM

A variety of histories may give rise to a suspicion of a primary neck problem including a fall on the neck while jumping, having reared up and fallen over backward, or having collided with another horse or solid object, thus sustaining neck trauma. The horse may have neck pain from having pulled backward while being tied up. The horse may have no history of trauma but have abnormal neck posture, swelling, a stiff neck, neck pain, or difficulties in lowering and raising the head. The horse may have a performance-related problem such as unwillingness to work on the bit, an unsteady head carriage, or abnormal head posture. Occasionally the horse may violently raise the head and neck under specific circumstances when ridden. A neck lesion should also be considered in a horse with forelimb lameness when pain cannot be localized to the limb. Subtle hindlimb gait abnormalities, such as a tendency to stumble, or loss of hindlimb power may be caused by a proprioceptive deficit without overt ataxia, reflecting a compressive lesion of the cervical spinal cord.

CLINICAL EXAMINATION

The shape of the neck is influenced both by the way in which the horse works and its conformation. If a horse carries the head and neck high, with the head somewhat extended, the ventral strap muscles tend to be abnormally well developed, resulting in a ewe-neck conformation. Many horses naturally bend more easily to the right than to the left or vice versa, and the muscles on the side of the neck, especially craniodorsally, are developed asymmetrically. Such asymmetry is particularly obvious if the neck is viewed from above by the rider. If a horse is excessively thin, then the cervical vertebrae become prominent and the caudodorsal neck region becomes dorsally concave, whereas in a fit, well-muscled horse that works regularly on the bit, this region is dorsally convex. Most stallions and many native pony breeds have a prominent dorsal convexity to the neck region, resulting in a cresty appearance. A horse that is excessively fat tends to lay down plaques of fat throughout the body, including the neck region, and this can be misinterpreted as abnormal neck swelling.

If a horse is particularly "thick through the jaw"—that is, has a large mandible—it is physically difficult to work on the bit (ie, flexing at the poll so that the front of the head is approximately vertical). Although neck pain can cause a reluctance to work on the bit, more common causes include rider-associated or training problems, mouth pain, forelimb or hindlimb lameness, and back pain. Some horses strongly resist the rider's aids to work on the bit, despite the absence of pain. The most obvious problem to a rider in extreme cases may be a horse throwing its head into the air violently when ridden, although this may not reflect neck pain, but pain elsewhere (**Fig. 1**). The use of artificial aids such as draw or running reins, which give the rider a mechanical advantage, may help to break a vicious cycle and encourage the horse to become more submissive and compliant. Similarly, work on the lunge line using a chambon (a device that runs from the girth via a headpiece to the bit rings) or a Pessoa (a device that runs around the horse's hindquarters via a surcingle to the bit rings) can encourage a horse to work in a correct outline and develop fitness and strength of the appropriate musculature. Working the horse in trot over appropriately spaced trotting poles can also help to encourage a horse to work in a correct outline, with a round and supple back.

A rider may complain of neck stiffness or difficulties in getting a horse to bend correctly in a circle. Although this may be caused by neck pain, neck stiffness may be a protective mechanism by the horse to avoid pain associated with lameness,

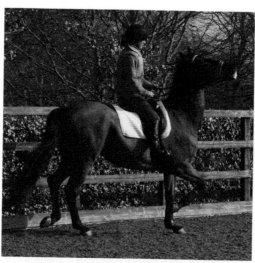

Fig. 1. An 8-year-old warmblood gelding had become difficult to ride, repeatedly throwing his head in the air. No clinical abnormalities were detected except when the horse was ridden. No overt lameness was detectable. Following perineural analgesia of the deep branch of the lateral plantar nerve of both hindlimbs, the horse worked with a normal neck posture. The horse had bilateral proximal suspensory desmitis. Abnormal neck posture does not necessarily reflect neck pain.

especially forelimb lameness. A horse with left forelimb lameness, for example, may be reluctant to bend properly to the left, and when unrestrained by a rider on the lunge, on the left rein may hold the neck and head slightly to the right, giving the appearance of looking out of the circle. Thus load distribution is altered and lameness minimized. Such lameness actually may not be evident during riding, although this may be the only circumstance under which the rider recognizes the performance problem. The lameness may be more obvious on the lunge or even in hand in straight lines. When a horse has an abnormal neck and/or head posture, a comprehensive clinical evaluation of the entire horse should be performed. Neck pain or abnormal posture may reflect a primary lesion elsewhere (eg, central or peripheral vestibular disease, fracture of the spinous processes of the cranial thoracic vertebrae, a mediastinal or thoracic abscess).

Detailed examination of the neck should include assessment of the neck conformation, the shape and posture at rest, and the position of the head relative to the neck and trunk. Patchy sweating or change in hair color reflecting intermittent sweating may suggest local damage to a sympathetic nerve as a branch of the nerve exits each vertebrae. Look carefully at the musculature to identify any localized atrophy. Palpate the right and left sides of the neck to assess symmetry and the presence of abnormal swellings or depressions and to identify any neck muscle pain (including reactive acupuncture points[1]), tension, hyperesthesia, analgesia, or fasciculation. Deep palpation should be performed on the left and right sides of the neck to identify pain and crepitation.

Neck flexibility should be assessed from side to side and up and down. This can be done by manually manipulating the neck, but many normal horses resist this. Holding a bowl of food by the horse's shoulder to assess lateral flexibility is helpful. Ideally the horse should be positioned against a wall, so that the horse cannot swing its

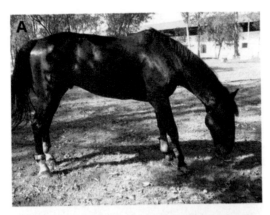

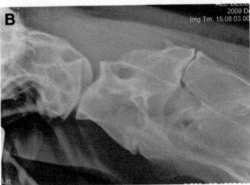

Fig. 2. (*A*) A 7-year-old warmblood gelding showing difficulty in lowering its head to graze. The owner complained of neck stiffness when ridden. The horse had congenital occipitoatlantoaxial malformation, and it is presumed that inability to extend the occipitoatlantoaxial articulations resulted in difficulties when grazing. (*B*) Lateral-lateral radiographic image of the cranial aspect of the neck of the horse in *A*. Cranial is to the left. The vertebrae are very abnormal in shape reflecting congenital occipitoatlantoaxial malformation. (*A* and *B, Courtesy of* Ana Stela Fonseca, DVM, Rio de Janeiro, Brazil.)

hindquarters away from the examiner during this assessment. The clinician should try to differentiate between the horse properly flexing the neck and twisting the head on the neck. Compare flexibility to the left and to the right. To assess extension of the neck, evaluate the ease with which the horse can stretch to eat from above head height. Observing the horse grazing is helpful to assess ventral mobility of the neck; the horse may find it difficult to lower the head to the ground (**Fig. 2**). Especially with lesions in the caudal neck region, a horse may have to straddle the forelimbs excessively to lower the head to the ground to graze. The horse should also be observed moving in small circles to the left and the right, and loose on the lunge.

Assessing skin sensation and local reflexes, such as the cervicofacial and the thoracolaryngeal reflexes, and comparing carefully the right and left sides may be useful. The consistency and patency of the jugular veins should be evaluated. Septic thrombophlebitis may cause neck stiffness.

The horse should be observed moving in hand and on the lunge, and if necessary should be ridden, to assess neck posture and the presence of neurologic gait abnormalities, restriction in forelimb gait, or lameness. The clinician should note how any gait abnormality is influenced by the positions of the head and neck. Forelimb lameness occasionally is associated with a primary cervical lesion, usually, but not invariably, together with other clinical signs referable to the neck.[2] Elevation of the head at a walk may result in enhanced scuffing of the front feet in horses with mild cervical compressive myelopathy.

DIAGNOSTIC IMAGING
Radiography and Radiology

Lateral-lateral radiographic images are obtained easily in the standing position; acquisition of images from left to right and right to left may be useful to determine the laterality of a lesion.[3] Lateral oblique images of the cervical vertebrae may give additional information concerning left-right symmetry of the APJs and axial extension of modeling changes.[4,5] Positioning of the neck is important, because any rotation of the head and neck makes it difficult to evaluate the APJs in particular. However, markedly asymmetric enlargement of caudal cervical APJs may make it impossible to obtain true lateral images of more cranial articulations.

A number of variations of the normal radiologic appearance of the cervical vertebrae should not be mistaken for lesions. A spur on the dorsocaudal aspect of the second cervical vertebral body may project dorsally into the vertebral canal. However, the vertebral canal has a large diameter at this site; therefore, spinal cord compromise is highly unlikely. The ventral processes of the sixth cervical vertebra and occasionally other vertebrae have small separate centers of ossification. The ventral lamina on the sixth cervical vertebra may be transposed onto the ventral aspect of the seventh cervical vertebra, unilaterally or bilaterally. The seventh cervical vertebra has a small spinous process, which may be superimposed over the APJs between the sixth and seventh cervical vertebrae and should not be confused with periarticular new bone. In older horses, small spondylitic spurs may be seen on the ventral aspect of the vertebral bodies. Modeling of the APJs between the fifth and sixth and between the sixth and seventh cervical vertebrae is common in middle-aged and older horses (**Fig. 3**).[3,6,7] An anatomic study of mature nonataxic horses revealed unilateral (53%) or bilateral (18%) overriding hyperextension arthropathy and buttressing of the APJs between the sixth and seventh cervical vertebrae (Katherine Whitwell, MRCVS, Newmarket, Suffolk, personal communication, June 2005). The modeling often is accompanied by extension of fibrocartilage across the cranial border of the dorsal arch of the seventh cervical vertebra and irregular enlargement of the articular processes.[6,7] The spinous process of the seventh cervical vertebra may become flattened or fragmented by contact with the sixth cervical vertebra when the neck is extended. Radiologically, these changes result in irregularity of the normally smooth outline of the APJs. A bony knob may develop on the ventral aspect of one or both cranial articular processes at the APJs between the fifth and sixth cervical vertebrae and between the sixth and seventh cervical vertebrae. When well developed, this knob forms a buttress that impinges onto the body or the arch of the more cranial vertebra and forms a false joint. The buttress partially obliterates the intervertebral foramen, but it is often of no clinical significance.[3,6,7] Buttresses occur at the APJs between the sixth and seventh cervical vertebrae in 18% of asymptomatic horses.[6] These modeling changes reflect the greatest range of motion of the most caudal cervical vertebrae. A recent radiologic study was performed using 122 sports horses and general purpose riding horses either with no clinical signs referable to the neck (n = 77), or with clinical signs related to lesions of the fifth and sixth cervical vertebrae (n = 45).[7] Radiographs of the caudal APJs of the cervical vertebrae were graded

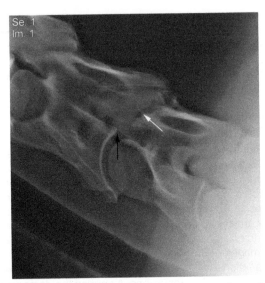

Fig. 3. Lateral-lateral radiographic image of the caudal aspect of a neck including the sixth cervical to first thoracic vertebrae. Cranial is to the left. There is marked asymmetric modeling of the APJs between the sixth and seventh cervical vertebrae (*white arrow*), with ventral buttressing (*black arrow*), and therefore marked narrowing of the intervertebral foramina.

objectively by 2 analysts. There was no significant association between discipline, breed, age, or clinical signs, although there was a trend for more severe lesions in older horses. The lack of association of grade with age may reflect both the relatively small size of the study population and the under representation of very young horses. Nonetheless the presence of abnormalities consistent with osteoarthritis is not synonymous with clinically significant lesions.

Major radiologic abnormalities such as fusion of two adjacent vertebrae can be present subclinically, in part because of the great mobility between adjacent vertebrae. The clinical significance of such lesions may also be determined by the athletic demands placed on the horse.

Nuclear Scintigraphy

Nuclear scintigraphy is a relatively insensitive technique for identification of neck lesions, and there are a high proportion of potentially false-positive results because in clinically normal horses there is usually greater radiopharmaceutical uptake (RU) in the bones of the APJs between the fifth and sixth and sixth and seventh cervical vertebrae, compared with the more cranial articulations reflecting the mobility of these joints[8,9] and the biomechanical forces imposed on these articulations.[10] Images should be obtained from the left and right sides because lesions may be uniaxial and are easily missed if images are obtained from the contralateral side. There is often greater RU in the odontoid peg (dens) of the axis, compared with the surrounding vertebrae. The shape of radiopharmaceutical distribution should be assessed carefully because a change in shape even without increased radiopharmaceutical uptake (IRU) may be important. Fractures are not always associated with prominent IRU, and lesions may be missed in the caudal neck region because of the overlying muscle mass resulting in shielding and the scapulae.

Diagnostic Ultrasonography

Ultrasonographic examination is useful for assessment of swellings, lesions of the ligamentum nuchae, the nuchal bursa, the intercentral and APJs, jugular vein thrombophlebitis, and for administering ultrasound-guided injections.[11–15]

Electromyography

Electromyography (EMG) can be used to quantify the motor unit action potential and to identify insertional activity and pathologic spontaneous electrical activity in muscle that can help to differentiate between myopathy and neuropathy and to localize the source of a lesion. It has been suggested that EMG can be used to help to determine the clinical significance of radiologic abnormalities of the cervical vertebrae by detection of evidence of neuropathy.[16]

MUSCLE LESIONS

The clinical significance of localized muscle soreness and/or tenseness is poorly understood and documented. I have had experience with a number of horses with subtle performance problems, including slight neck stiffness, reluctance to work properly on the bit and to accept an even contact, and intermittent, slight gait irregularities associated with soreness around and in front of the wings of the axis. Clinical improvement has been seen after relief of this pain by rapid and sudden rotation of the head about the axis.[17] There is also little doubt that some horses with focal muscle soreness in the neck show improved performance after physiotherapy or osteopathic treatment.

Many horses resent firm palpation of the brachiocephalicus muscles at the base of the neck. This may be more obvious in horses with forelimb lameness, especially those with pain in the distal part of the limb. This muscle soreness is generally a secondary rather than a primary cause of lameness. Transient improvement in gait may be seen after local therapy using laser therapy, H-wave therapy, TENS, therapeutic ultrasound, and/or massage.

Primary brachiocephalicus pain at the base of the neck has been seen in performance horses, causing subtle gait abnormalities at the walk when ridden, characterized by abnormal lifting of the neck as the limb was advanced and a shortened cranial phase of the stride ipsilateral to the sore muscle. Lameness may also be seen in trot when performing lateral work, such as half-pass in the direction away from the lame limb. Bilateral brachiocephalicus muscle pain has also been seen in association with throwing up of the head when in the air over a fence and on landing. Treatment of the sore muscles abolished this behavior.

Local muscle soreness also may be seen with a poorly fitting saddle or girth or with a rider who is unable to ride truly in balance with the horse. The primary problem must be addressed if treatment is to be successful. Some driving horses develop forelimb lameness that is seen only when the horse is pulling and may be associated with pressure from the harness, for example a collar. Adaptation of the harness may relieve the problem.

Some horses seem to need to learn how to use the neck and forelimb musculature to maximum advantage and have a restricted forelimb gait without appearing overtly lame. The gait is not altered by distal limb nerve blocks. Some improvement may be achieved by daily massage of the muscles at the base of the neck and manual full protraction of the forelimbs. This is combined with exercise to encourage the horse to lengthen the forelimb stride and to round the back. Lunging in a chambon or Pessoa, trotting over appropriately placed trot poles, and repeatedly lengthening and

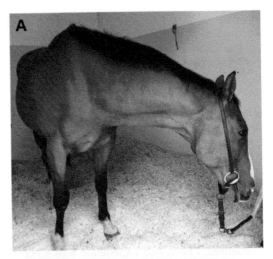

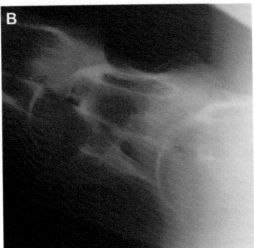

Fig. 4. (A) A 7-year-old warmblood gelding with the head and neck stuck in an abnormal posture with the neck held low and turned to the left. There was a dried patch of sweat on the caudal aspect of the right side of the neck. By careful manipulation of the neck, it could become "unlocked" with the horse immediately adopting a more normal posture. This was a sporadic occurrence. While the neck was stuck the horse was extremely reluctant to move. (B) Lateral-lateral radiographic image of the caudal aspect of the neck of the horse illustrated in A, including the fifth to seventh cervical vertebrae. Cranial is to the left. There is marked enlargement of the APJs between the fifth and sixth and sixth and seventh cervical vertebrae and narrowing of the intervertebral foramina with the potential to cause episodic nerve root impingement.

shortening the stride all may be beneficial. Trotting down the tramlines in a field of corn or rapeseed can also be of enormous help.

Occasionally as the result of a fall or pulling back when tied, acute severe neck muscle soreness develops. The horse is best treated initially with nonsteroidal anti-inflammatory drugs (NSAIDs), rest, and local physiotherapy, followed by progressive remobilization when the acute muscle soreness has subsided. The prognosis is good.

There is a syndrome of episodic transient attacks of profound neck pain and stiffness, with the horse holding the neck in a relatively low position (**Fig. 4**). In some horses, a severe unilateral forelimb lameness occurs, often resulting in the limb being held in a semiflexed position at rest. These attacks vary in duration (hours to days), and generally horses have been completely normal between episodes. To date, neither a definitive cause nor an effective treatment in the long term has been identified for this syndrome. However, there is usually a very marked enlargement of the caudal cervical APJs (see earlier and under Osteoarthritis), with narrowing of the intervertebral foramen, and it is suspected that nerve root impingement may cause episodic pain. Careful manipulation of the caudal neck region may result in instantaneous relief of clinical signs. It is difficult to determine whether medication of the APJs is of any benefit because of the sporadic and infrequent nature of the clinical signs in most affected horses. In North America similar signs may be seen in horses seropositive for *Borrelia burgdoferi* and those with a positive clinical response to Doxycycline therapy (T.J. Divers, personal communication, 2011).

INSERTIONAL DESMOPATHY OF THE NUCHAL LIGAMENT AND INJURY TO SEMISPINALIS

The nuchal ligament is a bilobed structure, fans at its insertion on the occiput, and is surrounded by muscle, the semispinalis to the left and right and the rectus capitis ventrally. New bone formation at the insertion on the occiput may be an incidental finding (**Fig. 5**). Examination of 302 warmbloods from 1 to 22 years of age revealed new bone in 85%. A postmortem study of warmbloods revealed a similar high proportion of horses with chondroid metaplasia at the insertion of the ligament and dystrophic mineralization.[17] A smaller radiologic study of thoroughbreds revealed new bone on the caudal aspect of the occiput in only 5%.[17]

Horses with insertional desmopathy of the nuchal ligament or injury to the tendon of insertion of semispinalis often have a history of trauma to the region (eg, pulling back when tied up) or an excessive amount of lunging exercise while restricted with side or draw reins.[17–19] Horses should be examined while being lunged, with and without side reins, and ridden. Clinical signs include permanent resistance against the reins, with difficulty or unwillingness to lower and flex the head and neck when ridden and poor flexion at the poll. In contrast to horses with back pain, hindlimb impulsion is usually good. The horse may have a tendency to rear or shake its head.

Pain cannot usually be elicited by palpation. Radiologic examination may reveal new bone on the caudal aspect of the occiput that may extend farther ventrally and dorsally than the actual insertion of the ligamentum nuchae. Mineralization sometimes is seen dorsal to the first cervical vertebra as an incidental radiologic finding, unassociated with clinical signs. Scintigraphic examination findings may be negative. Ultrasonographic examination is not easy, and interpretation is difficult. Mineralization within the ligament may cause shadowing artifacts. CT offers the most sensitive means of detecting lesions in either the nuchal ligaments or the border of insertion of semispinalis.[17–19] Diagnosis depends on a positive response to infiltration of local anesthetic solution. Fifteen milliliters of mepivacaine is infiltrated on the left and right sides, and the response is assessed after 15 to 30 minutes. Care must be taken not to inject into the epidural space, which will result in ataxia.

Treatment consists of repeated infiltration of corticosteroids, traumeel (a homeopathic remedy), and local anesthetic solution and modification of the training program, with no work on the bit for 8 weeks.[19] The horse should be worked principally in straight lines. In the stable the horse should be encouraged to flex the poll region gently from side to side and up and down. The use of acupuncture or magnetic field therapy, laser

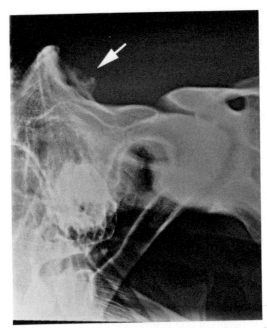

Fig. 5. Lateral-lateral radiographic image of the cranial aspect of the neck of a horse. Cranial is to the left. There is an exostosis in the caudal aspect of the occiput. This is a common incidental abnormality.

therapy, ultrasound, or shock wave therapy may help some horses. The results vary. Seventy percent of 26 horses returned to full work, although not all were completely normal. Extracorporeal shock wave therapy, two or three applications at 14-day intervals, in addition to 4 weeks of work without requiring flexion of the poll, has been reported to be successful in resolving clinical signs in 12 of 22 horses and in improving signs in 6 other horses.[20] Surgical treatment by transection of the nuchal ligament and the fascia of semispinalis has resulted in improvement in a small number of horses refractory to conservative management (Michael Nowak, Germany, personal communication, 2004).

NUCHAL BURSITIS

A rare cause of neck stiffness, pain, or abnormal neck posture is noninfectious or infectious bursitis.[15] There may be localized soft tissue swelling, but diagnosis is dependent on ultrasonographic identification of a distended bursa dorsal to the first and second cervical vertebrae. Surgical debridement has resulted in resolution of clinical signs.

SUBLUXATION OF THE FIRST AND SECOND CERVICAL VERTEBRAE

Subluxation of the first and second cervical vertebrae is an unusual condition, probably related to trauma such as a fall, although the horse may have no recent history of such.[21–26] The condition is associated with damage of the ligament of the dens or the ventral longitudinal ligament between the first and second cervical vertebrae or occurs secondary to a fracture of the dens.[22,23] An affected horse usually has a stiff neck and a tendency for the head and neck to be somewhat extended. Differentiating between neck pain and stiffness may be difficult. An audible clicking noise may emanate from the region, and occasionally abnormal movement between the vertebrae can be appreciated. Because of the relatively wide sagittal diameter of the vertebral canal at this site, generally no associated compression of the cervical spinal cord occurs. Occasionally, neurologic abnormalities are seen in horses with a displaced fracture of the dens.[26]

Diagnosis is based on radiologic examination, using lateral-lateral images with the neck in natural (neutral) and extended positions. Radiologic abnormalities may include abnormal orientation between the first and second cervical vertebrae. The position of the dens may be abnormal, resulting in narrowing of the space between it and the dorsal lamina of the vertebral arch of the first cervical vertebra. In a study of yearling thoroughbreds, the mean minimum sagittal diameter was 34 mm and the minimum was 26 mm.[27] Narrowing of the distance between the vertebral arch of the first and second cervical vertebrae may occur in an extended versus neutral position of the neck. The shape of the dens may be altered because of secondary new bone formation. Occasionally, the dens is fractured, usually at the junction between the odontoid process and the body of the vertebra.[26]

Acute fractures of the dens occur occasionally resulting in neck pain and ataxia. Four of five horses with an acute fracture of the dens returned to athletic function, despite neurologic gait abnormalities at the time of acute injury, although one had a tendency to trip.[26]

Congenital occipitoatlantoaxial malformation is usually recognized in foals because of obvious abnormality in shape of the cranial aspect of the neck. Occasionally however this may be recognized in an older horse with a stiff neck (**Fig. 2B**).

SUBLUXATION OF THE FIFTH AND SIXTH OR SIXTH AND SEVENTH CERVICAL VERTEBRAE

Subluxation of the fifth and sixth or sixth and seventh cervical vertebrae is usually recognized in adult horses with a complaint of lack of hindlimb power or with difficulties in performing movements requiring collection or, if a breeding stallion, difficulties in mounting either mares or a dummy. Careful clinical examination usually reveals mild-to-moderate hindlimb ataxia, although this has not generally been recognized by the owner. Such horses may have an extravagant gait but rarely have the power or coordination to perform at a high level. Radiologic examination reveals either dorsal or less commonly ventral displacement of the head of the sixth or seventh cervical vertebra (**Fig. 6**). Subluxation of the sixth and seventh cervical vertebrae has less commonly been identified as a cause of bilateral forelimb lameness.[28]

OSTEOARTHRITIS OF THE CERVICAL ARTICULAR PROCESS JOINTS

The potential exists for large amounts of new bone associated with osteoarthritis of the cervical APJs to encroach axially into the vertebral canal, resulting in compression of the spinal cord and hindlimb weakness and ataxia, or into the intervertebral foramen, resulting in nerve root compression with local or referred pain and possibly lameness and patchy sweating. Thickening of the joint capsule and ligamentum flavum and synovial cyst formation may contribute. Resultant neurogenic muscle atrophy may alter forelimb support and change functional gait. Dermatomal sweating is thought to be due to impingement on the vertebral sympathetic nerve (or its branches), which runs alongside the vertebral artery in the paravertebral foramina. Branches of the vertebral nerve are thought to join the spinal nerve roots as they

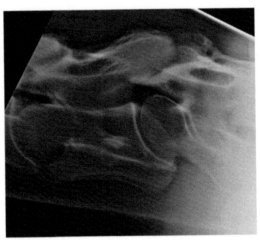

Fig. 6. Lateral-lateral radiographic image of the sixth and seventh cervical vertebrae of a 6-year-old thoroughbred cross warmblood event horse gelding with a history of poor performance. The horse showed low-grade hindlimb ataxia. Cranial is to the left. There is marked subluxation of the intercentral articulation, with dorsal displacement of the head of the seventh cervical vertebra. The vertebral canal of the seventh cervical vertebra is wedge-shaped, being narrower cranially. There is asymmetric enlargement of the APJs consistent with osteoarthritis.

leave the intervertebral foramen providing autonomic fibers locally.[28] Local cervical reflexes may be reduced or absent resulting in an area of hypoaesthesia. Local hyperesthesia has also been reported in association with cervical vertebral compressive myelopathy.[29] Severe osteoarthritic change may progress to partial or complete fusion and thus neck stiffness.

Radiologic abnormalities associated with osteoarthritis include enlargement of one or more of the APJs and alteration in joint space width (see **Fig. 3**; **Figs. 4**B, and **7**). Widening of the joint space is usually associated with asymmetric facet enlargement; narrowing is caused by articular cartilage degeneration. Pitted lucent zones may develop in the articular facets, with extension of the dorsal laminae between adjacent vertebrae and partial or complete obliteration of the adjacent intervertebral foramina. Sometimes fractures are seen dorsal to a joint. Abnormalities often develop on both the left and right sides but are frequently asymmetric. With substantial asymmetry of the APJs, the affected and immediately more cranial vertebrae may appear rotated on a lateral radiographic image, although the horse had appeared to be standing with its head and neck straight in the sagittal plane. Radiographic examination from left to right and from right to left and oblique radiographic projections can help to determine on which side a unilateral lesion is present. A lesion that is close to the imaging plate is clearer and magnification is less than if the lesion is on the opposite side of the neck. Ultrasonography can also be used to demonstrate periarticular modeling and synovial effusion.

The clinical importance of osteoarthritis of one or more APJs can be difficult to determine by clinical and radiologic examinations alone, except by exclusion. The greater the degree of abnormality and the larger the number of articulations involved, the more likely the condition is clinically significant. In normal horses, finding osteoarthritic change cranial to the APJs between the fifth and sixth cervical vertebrae

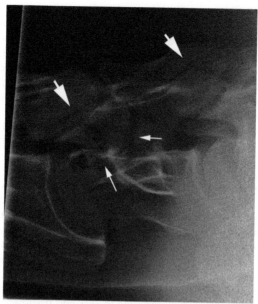

Fig. 7. Lateral-lateral radiographic image of the sixth cervical to first thoracic vertebrae of a 6-year-old Irish sport horse gelding. Cranial is to the left. The horse had sudden onset of profound ataxia 2 days previously, but retrospectively had become stiffer in the neck and less willing to work consistently on the bit over the previous several months. There was marked pain in the caudal neck region, especially on the right side. There is asymmetric enlargement of the APJs of the sixth and seventh cervical vertebrae and the seventh cervical and first thoracic vertebrae, consistent with osteoarthritis (*arrowheads*). There is a nondisplaced fracture through the pedicle of the seventh thoracic vertebra with mild increased opacity along the margins of the fracture (*arrows*). Postmortem examination confirmed spinal cord compression at this site. The fracture was clearly chronic but unstable.

is relatively rare. Unilateral forelimb lameness has been seen with lesions between the fourth cervical and first thoracic vertebrae.[2] Nuclear scintigraphic examination may give further information in horses with neck stiffness or forelimb lameness apparently not referable to the limb itself. Ultrasound-guided intra-articular analgesia or medication may help to determine the significance of radiologic abnormalities. A dorsal approach is recommended for intra-articular analgesia.[13,14]

In one report, 7 of 8 horses with forelimb lameness associated with radiologic abnormalities of the cervical vertebrae also had subtle to obvious signs of neck pain.[2] Patterns of muscle atrophy in the neck and shoulder regions varied. The character of the lameness varied. Radiologic abnormalities included substantial modeling of the APJs in the caudal neck region in 3 horses; a fourth had modeling and a fracture involving the APJs between the fourth and fifth cervical vertebrae. One horse had abnormalities of the intercentral articulation between the seventh cervical and first thoracic vertebrae and a discrete mineralized fragment dorsal to it. Large lucent zones were identified in a vertebral body (the fourth and sixth cervical vertebrae) in 2 horses. A fracture of the vertebral body of the seventh cervical vertebra was seen in 1 horse.

An additional 7 horses examined at the Animal Health Trust between 1994 and 2009 with forelimb lameness and no ataxia were thought to have forelimb lameness associated with advanced osteoarthritis of the APJs between the fifth cervical and first thoracic vertebrae. An additional 2 horses had asymmetrically enlarged APJs of the sixth and seventh synovial articulations and a fracture through one of the articular processes of the seventh cervical vertebra. All horses had undergone a full orthopedic assessment, complete analgesic techniques of the lame forelimb, and radiologic assessment of the shoulder and elbow joints and cranial ribs. Gait changes included a lowered arc of foot flight, shortened cranial phase of stride, and moving with the neck held stiffly and/or extended in 2 horses. In 4 horses, lameness was more marked when ridden compared with in hand and on the lunge, with the lame forelimb on the outside of a circle. Ultrasound-guided intra-articular analgesia of the affected facet joints was performed in 4 horses, all of which showed partial improvement in lameness. Nuclear scintigraphic examination was unhelpful in confirming the diagnosis in the 5 horses in which it was performed.

Nerve root impingement in the caudal neck may cause radicular or referred pain and account for forelimb lameness. Neck pain itself can also cause forelimb lameness. Compression of the seventh cervical nerve was confirmed postmortem in a horse with osteoarthritis of the APJs between the sixth and seventh cervical vertebrae and between the seventh cervical and first thoracic vertebrae.[2] Nerve root compression in association with severe osteoarthritis has also been demonstrated using contrast-enhanced CT.[30]

In horses with mild ataxia, neck stiffness, or forelimb lameness associated with osteoarthritis of cervical APJs, the response to rest and treatment with NSAIDs has been limited. Local periarticular or intra-articular infiltration of corticosteroids, performed using ultrasonographic guidance, may bring temporary relief. There is limited documented evidence for the efficacy and duration of effect of medication of the APJs of the caudal cervical vertebrae. In a recent study of 59 sports or pleasure horses with ataxia, neck stiffness or pain, or obscure forelimb lameness, 19 horses (32%) returned to full function and 18 horses (31%) improved more than 50%.[31] However, the effect was generally short lived, with 55% showing improvement for a duration of less than 1 month to up to 6 months. The inclusion criteria for the study were poorly defined and follow-up results were based on the owners' subjective opinions. Injection of the APJs was described in 150 horses, the majority of which showed poor performance, lameness, neck stiffness, or neck pain, but the response to treatment was not documented.[32] Epidural injection of corticosteroids performed with the horse under general anesthesia has been shown to result in relief of neck stiffness in a horse with osteoarthritis of the APJs between the fourth and fifth cervical vertebrae and clinical evidence of nerve root compression.[33]

Osteoarthritis, especially in the caudal neck region, may result in associated enlargement of the joint capsule(s), the development of a synovial hernia and subsequent pressure on the spinal cord. In horses with mild osteoarthritis obvious ataxia may not be seen, but the history may include the tendency to stumble or to knuckle behind, or lack of hindlimb impulsion. Such signs often have been attributed to lameness but are invariably unaltered by diagnostic treatment with NSAIDs. Clinical signs may be subtle and intermittent. Such horses usually show abnormal weakness if pulled to one side by traction on the tail while the horse is walking—the sway test. A normal horse easily may be pulled off line once, but then strongly resists. A weak horse can be pulled off line repeatedly. Weakness may also be apparent as the horse decelerates from trot to walk, with exaggerated up-and-down movement of the hindquarters and asymmetric hindlimb placement. This may result in irregular movement of each patella and may be confused with mild intermittent upward fixation or delayed release of the patella. At faster speeds, the horse may look completely normal, although some affected horses demonstrate a remarkably croup-high canter when on the lunge. In a young horse, advanced osteoarthritis of one or more caudal cervical APJs is strong circumstantial evidence of cause and effect. Definitive diagnosis in an older horse is much more difficult, because radiologic evidence of osteoarthritis may be present without associated clinical signs. Myelography may help but false positive and negative results occur.[34,35] With moderate to severe clinical signs the prognosis is poor, and affected horses may be potentially unsafe to ride. Horses with mild clinical signs (grade ≤2/5 ataxia) may show improvement after intra-articular medication of affected APJs with triamcinolone (8 mg) or methyl prednisolone acetate (40 mg), with up to 80% of horses showing resolution of clinical signs from 1 to 3 months after treatment for up to 2 to 3 years (Richard Hepburn MRCVS, Gloucestershire, personal communication, December 2010). Surgical treatment can be considered and generally results in clinical improvement, but few sports horses become upper-level athletes, and some develop recurrent ataxia several years later.

DISKOSPONDYLITIS

A survey of the cervical intervertebral disks of 103 horses from birth to 23 years of age confirmed that they consisted solely of fibrocartilage, with no nucleus pulposus.[36] Age-related degenerative changes were identified, but even with severe disintegration of the disks, no referable clinical signs had been apparent. However, disk degeneration and dorsal bulging of the dorsal longitudinal ligament may increase intervertebral mobility and could potentially contribute to spinal nerve root compression (Katherine Whitwell, MRCVS, Newmarket, Suffolk, personal communication, December 2010).

Diskospondylitis is a rare cause of neck pain, forelimb lameness, or ataxia.[37–39] Although diskospondylitis is usually an infectious condition in dogs, no proved relationship occurs in the adult horse, and trauma may be an inciting cause. Lesions in the horse have been identified in the caudal neck region (the articulations between the sixth and seventh cervical vertebrae and the seventh cervical and first thoracic vertebrae) and between the third and fourth cervical vertebrae in association with severe neck pain and a bilaterally short, stiff forelimb lameness or episodic, unilateral forelimb lameness (**Fig. 8**). Occasionally a horse may be reluctant to work "on the bit" but shows no other detectable clinical signs. High-quality radiographs are required for accurate diagnosis. Lesions are characterized by loss of the normal opacity of the cranial and caudal endplates of the affected vertebrae, with or without alteration in the intercentral joint space. Scintigraphic examination may help to localize the affected joint(s). The prognosis is guarded, although in one report a broodmare that was admitted with profound neck pain and periodic severe left forelimb lameness, associated with irregularity of the endplates at the intercentral articulation between the sixth and seventh cervical vertebrae and narrowing of the intercentral space, after a collision with a fence, made a spontaneous recovery.[37] A second horse was treated by surgical debridement of the disc space and implantation of a cancellous bone graft, with resolution of clinical signs.

Radiologic recognition of discospondylitis at the cervicothoracic junction has occasionally been seen unassociated with definitive clinical signs of either lameness or abnormal neck posture.

FRACTURES OF THE CERVICAL VERTEBRAE

Fractures of the cervical vertebrae usually result from trauma: the horse rearing up and falling over backward or sideways; pulling back when tied up; or falling while

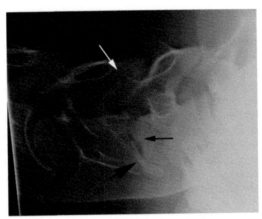

Fig. 8. Lateral-lateral radiographic image of the sixth cervical to second thoracic vertebrae of a 5-year-old pony gelding with left forelimb lameness and extreme difficulties in lowering the head to the ground to graze. Cranial is to the left. There is marked asymmetric enlargement of the APJs of the seventh cervical and first thoracic vertebrae consistent with osteoarthritis (*white arrow*). The intercentral articulation between the seventh cervical and thoracic vertebrae is highly abnormal (*black arrows*). There is a concave radiolucent defect in the head of the first thoracic vertebra and discontinuity of the caudal end plate of the seventh cervical vertebra, with loss of the normal narrow radiopaque line, but with generalized increased opacity ventrally. The intercentral joint space is markedly narrowed consistent with discospondylitis. Ultrasound guided intra-articular analgesia of the left APJ between the seventh cervical and first thoracic vertebrae resulted in resolution of the left forelimb lameness and the pony was easily able to lower its head to graze. (*Courtesy of* Annamaria Nagy, DVM, MRCVS, Newmarket, Suffolk, England.)

jumping, usually at speed. Clinical signs are sudden in onset and include holding the neck in an abnormally low position, stiffness, a focal or more diffuse area of pain, with or without localized or more diffuse soft tissue swelling, and muscle guarding. Audible or palpable crepitus is sometimes detected. The horse may be unable to lower its head to the ground or may be able to do so only by straddling of the forelimbs. Associated hindlimb and forelimb ataxia may be apparent, which can be transient and self-resolving, or persistent. Patchy sweating and localized muscle atrophy may develop. Occasionally, an associated unilateral or bilateral forelimb lameness occurs.

Diagnosis is confirmed radiologically. Most fractures are detectable on lateral-lateral images, although lateral oblique and ventrodorsal images can also be helpful in selected horses. Care should be taken not to confuse physes and separate centers of ossification with fractures.

The prognosis depends on the site and configuration of the fracture(s), the degree of displacement, and hence the likelihood of permanent compression of the spinal cord, either by a displaced fracture or by subsequent callus formation.

Fractures of the atlas and axis, especially through the physis of the separate center of ossification of the dens, are particularly common in foals. The prognosis for complete recovery is fair with conservative management, provided that no evidence of ataxia exists. Usually no treatment is required other than confinement to a box or small pen.

Fractures of the cervical vertebrae in adults more commonly involve the vertebral body or arch in the mid-neck region (the third to sixth cervical vertebrae) or the APJs of the more caudal vertebrae (the fifth to seventh cervical vertebrae). Local hemorrhage and edema may result in ataxia, which usually resolves within a few days. Persistence of ataxia warrants a guarded prognosis. Most fractures heal by callus formation, and this may subsequently impinge on the spinal cord, causing later ataxia. A fracture of a vertebral body also may result in damage to the adjacent intervertebral disk and associated ligaments, which subsequently may protrude into the vertebral canal and cause ataxia. Thus, in the acute stage, giving an accurate prognosis may be difficult. However, many fractures of the vertebral bodies and APJs do heal, and horses may be able to return to athletic function, although residual neck stiffness may be present.

In the acute stage, the horse should be confined to box rest. Analgesics may be necessary to control severe pain, but they should be used judiciously to avoid encouraging excessive movement of the neck. The position of the water bucket and manger should be adjusted so that the horse can drink and eat from normal head height. The hay should be fed at a height level with the head, preferably loose, or if in a hay net, a net with large holes, with the hay well shaken first. The horse should not be tied up during the convalescent period in case it pulls back. Reappraising the horse clinically and radiologically every 6 to 8 weeks is helpful. Maximum clinical improvement may not be seen until 6 to 9 months after injury. Selected fractures may require surgical stabilization.[40]

MYELOMA

Myeloma is a myeloproliferative disorder that can cause radiolucent lesions in any bone, including the cervical vertebrae, with associated bone pain.[17,41,42] Cervical vertebral myeloma was diagnosed in several horses of a wide range of breeds and ages.[41] Differential diagnosis should include vertebral osteomyelitis or other primary or metastatic neoplasia, including hemangiosarcoma, osteosarcoma, chondrosarcoma, undifferentiated sarcoma, and malignant melanoma. Clinical signs included intermittent pyrexia, severe neck pain and stiffness, episodic forelimb lameness, weight loss, and a variety of other abnormalities. Diagnosis is based on hematologic, radiologic, and bone biopsy examinations. Hematologic abnormalities include anemia, leukocytosis, neutrophilia, and lymphocytosis. Total protein concentration is elevated greatly. Protein electrophoresis shows a monoclonal peak in the gamma region. Radiologic examination of affected bones reveals clearly demarcated lucent zones, usually without a rim of more radiopaque bone. Bone biopsy is useful to confirm the diagnosis, but currently no treatment is available and the prognosis is hopeless.

OTHER CYSTLIKE LESIONS IN CERVICAL VERTEBRAE

Occasionally, single or several well-demarcated radiolucent zones are identified in one or more adjacent vertebrae, associated with profound neck pain, with or without forelimb lameness. These lesions have not been proved to be caused by osteomyelitis or myeloma, although a definitive diagnosis has not always been possible by bone biopsy or postmortem examination. One horse with extremely severe neck pain and forelimb lameness had radiolucent zones in the fifth and sixth cervical vertebrae, and bone biopsy revealed accumulation of abnormal plasma cells, but the horse made a most spectacular and complete recovery after exploratory surgery and returned to international showjumping. A show pony had a large cystlike lesion in the fourth cervical vertebra with profound neck pain and left forelimb lameness. Postmortem examination revealed a cavity filled with granulation tissue, surrounded by a large area of bone necrosis, but no suggestion of the underlying cause.

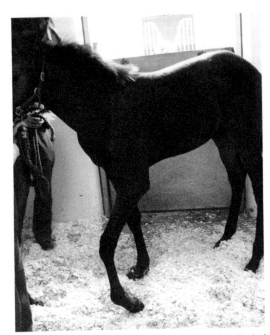

Fig. 9. A 5-month-old thoroughbred colt with marked left forelimb lameness of 5 days' duration and abnormal posture suggestive of radial nerve paralysis but accompanied also by instability of the shoulder and developing contracture of the carpus and fetlock. There was electromyographic evidence of both radial and ulnar nerve dysfunction. There was a fracture of the most proximal aspect of the first rib with associated damage of the eighth cervical nerve, which is a major contributor to the brachial plexus.

LESIONS OF THE FIRST RIB AND FORELIMB LAMENESS

Occasionally, unilateral forelimb lameness and odd patterns of muscle atrophy and abnormal forelimb posture have been identified in association with injury of the proximal aspect of the first rib and secondary damage to the eighth cervical nerve (**Fig. 9**). The posture may mimic radial nerve paralysis, but the pattern of muscle atrophy and other gait abnormalities are inconsistent with this. Electromyography can be useful for determining evidence of nerve damage to both the radial and ulnar nerves.

Several horses have been seen with acute traumatic fractures of the first rib and ipsilateral forelimb lameness.[17] A variety of congenital abnormalities of the first rib have been identified in association with unexplained forelimb lameness (Dyson, S., unpublished data; Katherine Whitwell, MRCVS, Newmarket, Suffolk, personal communication, March 2007; Mike Ross, Kennett Square, Pennsylvania, personal communication, July 2008). A 4-year-old thoroughbred mare had chronic right forelimb lameness, characterized by a marked shortened cranial phase of the stride, which did not respond to local analgesia. Radiologic examination revealed bilateral partial fusion of the first 2 ribs ventrally. At the junction of the proximal two-thirds of the first rib with the fused first and second ribs, there was evidence of a chronic nonunion fracture with extensive callus formation on the right side. Postmortem examination revealed a tough fibrous sheet of tissue extending between the callus and the axial aspect of the shoulder joint, within which was a fluid-filled cavity through which some of the nerves of the brachial plexus passed. It was speculated that nerve entrapment and neuralgia may have caused pain.

BORRELIA BURGDORFERI AND ASSOCIATION WITH NERVE ROOT LESIONS

Borrelia burgdorferi infection has anecdotally been associated with shifting limb lameness and other clinical signs possibly attributable to cervical nerve root pathology. However, there is a high frequency of high antibody titers in horses in tick-infested areas and specificity of antibody titer for clinical disease is therefore low. However, histologic examination has revealed lymphocytic infiltration of nerve roots and a positive PCR assay for *Borrelia burgdorferi* (Tom Divers, DVM, Ithaca, NY, personal communication, July 2009). A horse with neck stiffness and central neurologic signs had a positive PCR assay for *Borrellia burgdoferi* DNA in cerebrospinal fluid and postmortem evidence of peripheral radiculoneuritis attributed to borrelliosis.[43]

SUMMARY

Lesions of the neck are an uncommon primary cause of pain resulting in either lameness or poor performance but should be considered if local analgesic techniques of the limbs fail to abolish lameness or if there are clinical signs directly referable to the neck such as pain, abnormal neck posture, stiffness, or patchy sweating. Accurate diagnosis requires careful clinical examination, exclusion of other causes of lameness or poor performance, and accurate interpretation of diagnostic imaging findings.

REFERENCES

1. Panzer R. Traditional Chinese veterinary medical diagnostics. In: Colahan P, Mayhew I, Merritt A, et al, editors. Equine medicine and surgery. 5th edition. St. Louis, MO: Mosby; 1999.
2. Ricardi G, Dyson S. Forelimb lameness associated with radiographic abnormalities of the cervical vertebrae. Equine Vet J 1993;25:422–6.
3. Butler J, Colles C, Dyson S, et al. The spine. In: Clinical radiology of the horse. 3rd edition. Oxford, UK: Wiley-Blackwell; 2008. p. 505–72.
4. Withers J, Voûte, L, Hammond G, et al. Radiographic anatomy of the articular process joints of the caudal cervical vertebrae in the horse on lateral and oblique projections. Equine Vet J 2009;41:895–902.
5. Dimock A, Puchalski S. Cervical radiology. Equine Vet Educ 2010;22:83–7.
6. Whitwell K, Dyson S. Interpreting radiographs. VIII. Equine cervical vertebrae. Equine Vet J 1987;19:8–14.
7. Down S, Henson F. A radiographic retrospective study of the caudal cervical articular process joints in the horse. Equine Vet J 2009;41:518–24.
8. Dyson S, Pilsworth R, Twardock R, et al. Equine scintigraphy. Equine Vet J 2003.
9. Didierlaurent V, Contremoulins V, Denoix H-M, et al. Scintigraphic pattern of uptake of [99m]technetium by the cervical vertebrae of sound horses. Vet Rec 2009;164:809–13.
10. Clayton M, Townsend H. Kinematics of the cervical spine in the adult horse. Equine Vet J 1989;21:189–92.
11. Gardner S, Reef V, Spencer P. Ultrasonographic evaluation of horses with thrombophlebitis of the jugular vein: 46 cases (1985-1988). J Am Vet Med Assoc 1991;199: 370–3.
12. Berg L, Nielsen J, Thoefner M, et al. Ultrasonography of the equine cervical region: a descriptive study in eight horses. Equine Vet J 2003;35:647–55.

13. Nielsen J, Berg L, Thoefner M, et al. Accuracy of ultrasound-guided intra-articular injection of cervical facet joints in horses: a cadaveric study. Equine Vet J 2003;35: 657–61.

14. Matoon J, Drost W, Weisbrode S. Technique for equine cervical articular process joint injection. Vet Radiol Ultrasound 2004;45:238–40.

15. Garcia-Lopez J, Jenei T, Chope K, et al. Diagnosis and management of cranial and caudal nuchal bursitis in four horses. J Am Vet Med Assoc 2010;237:823–9.

16. Wijnberg I, Back W, de Jong M, et al. The role of electromyography in clinical diagnosis of neuromuscular locomotor problems in the horse. Equine Vet J 2004;36: 718–22.

17. Dyson S. The cervical spine and soft tissues of the neck. In: Ross M, Dyson S, editors. Diagnosis and management of lameness in the horse. 2nd edition. St. Louis, MO: Elsevier; 2010. p. 606–16.

18. Nowak M, Huskamp B. Uber einige spezielle befunde bei erkrankungen der halswirbelsaule des pferdes. Pferdheilkunde 1989;5:95–107.

19. Nowak M. Die insertiondesmopathie des nackenstrangursprungs beim pferd. Diagnostik, differential diagnostik. Proceedings of the 7th Congress on Equine Medicine and Surgery, Geneva, 2001.

20. McClure S, Weinberger T. Extracorporeal shock wave therapy: clinical applications and regulation. Clin Tech Equine Pract 2003;2:358–67.

21. Funk K, Erikson E. Case report. A case of atlanto-axial subluxation in a horse. Can Vet J 1968;9:120–3.

22. Guffy M, Coffman J, Strafuss A. Atlantoaxial luxation in a foal. J Am Vet Med Assoc 1969;155:754–7.

23. Owen R, Smith-Maxie L. Repair of fractured dens of the axis in a foal. J Am Vet Med Assoc 1978;173:854–6.

24. McCoy D, Shires P, Beadle R. Ventral approach for stabilization of atlantoaxial subluxation secondary to odontoid fracture in a foal. J Am Vet Med Assoc 1984;185: 545–9.

25. Slone D, Bergfeld W, Walker T. Surgical decompression for traumatic atlantoaxial subluxation in a weanling filly. J Am Vet Med Assoc 1979;174:1234–6.

26. Vos N, Pollock P, Harty M, et al. Fractures of the cervical odontoid in four horses and one pony. Vet Rec 2008;162:116–9.

27. Mayhew I, Whitlock R, de Lahunta A. Spinal cord disease in the horse. Cornell Vet 1978;6(Suppl):13–207.

28. Mayhew J. Vertebral and paravertebral problems. In: Large animal neurology. 2nd edition. Oxford (UK): Wiley-Blackwell; 2009.

29. Levine J, Scrivani P, Divers T, et al. Multicenter case-control study of signalmen, diagnostic features, and outcome associated with cervical vertebral malformation-malarticulation in horses. J Am Vet Med Assoc 2010;237:812–22.

30. Moore B, Holbrook T, Stefanacci J, et al. Contrast-enhanced computed tomography and myelography in six horses with cervical stenotic myelopathy. Equine Vet J 1992;24:197–202.

31. Birmingham A, Reed S, Mattoon J, et al. Qualitative assessment of corticosteroid cervical articular facet injection in symptomatic horses. Equine Vet Educ 2010;22: 77–82.

32. Martinelli M, Rantanen N, Grant B. Cervical arthropathy, myelopathy or just a pain in the neck? Equine Vet Educ 2010;22:88–9.

33. Marks D. Cervical nerve root compression in a horse, treated by epidural injection of corticosteroid. J Equine Vet Sci 1999;19:399–401.

34. Butler J, Colles C, Dyson S, et al. Miscellaneous techniques. In: Clinical radiology of the horse. 3rd edition. Oxford (UK): Wiley-Blackwell; 2008. p. 685–709.
35. Van Biervliet J, Scrivani P, Divers T. Evaluation of decision criteria for detection of spinal cord compression based on cervical myelography in horses: 38 cases. Equine Vet J 2004;36:14–20.
36. Bollwein A, Hanichen T. Age related changes in the intervertebral disks of the cervical vertebral column in the horse. Tierarztl Prax 1989;17:73–6.
37. Adams S, Steckel R, Blevins W. Diskospondylitis in five horses. J Am Vet Med Assoc 1985;186:270–2.
38. Sweers L, Carstend A. Imaging features of discospondylitis in two horses. Vet Radiol Ultrasound 2006;47:159–64.
39. Speltz M, Olson E, Hunt L, et al. Equine intervertebral disk disease: a case report. J Equine Vet Sci 2006;26:413–9.
40. Barnes H, Tucker R, Grant B, et al. Lag screw stabilization of a cervical vertebral fracture by use of computed tomography in a horse. J Am Vet Med Assoc 1995;206:221–3.
41. MacAllister C, Qualls C, Tyler R, et al. Multiple myeloma in a horse. J Am Vet Med Assoc 1987;191:337–9.
42. Markel M, Dorr T. Multiple myeloma in a horse. J Am Vet Med Assoc 1986;188:621–3.
43. James F, Engiles J, Beech J. Meningitis, cranial neuritis and radiculoneuritis associated with Borrelia burgdorferi infection in a horse. J Am Vet Med Assoc 2010;237:1180–5.

Advanced Imaging of the Nervous System in the Horse

Peter V. Scrivani, DVM

KEYWORDS

- Computed tomography • Magnetic resonance imaging
- Radiography • Horse • Neurology

Neuroimaging is a branch of medical imaging that includes all methods for obtaining structural and functional images of a patient's nervous system including the brain, spinal cord, peripheral nervous system, and supporting soft and hard tissues. Structural imaging refers to the production of images that depict anatomy. Functional imaging refers to the production of images that depict physiologic activities such as changes in metabolism, blood flow, cerebrospinal fluid (CSF) flow, or regional chemical composition or diffusion of water protons.[1] Neurologic disease may produce morphologic changes, physiologic changes, or both. In veterinary medicine, the majority of neuroimaging is based on identifying morphologic changes.

In the past few decades, several advances have propelled neuroimaging forward including exquisite imaging capability for both patient morphology and function, better methods for distributing information, improved understanding of pathogenesis, and new paradigms for interpreting imaging examinations. Some of the most salient technical advances are new methods for examining the body (eg, multislice computed tomography [CT], high-field magnetic resonance imaging [MRI]), digitization of all imaging modalities, and the development of Radiology Information Systems (RIS), and Picture Archiving and Communications Systems (PACS) for efficient storage and distribution of medical images. These advances, combined with new treatment options, have greatly improved patient care for many individuals with neurologic disease.

Equine neuroimaging is a highly specialized field due to the rarity of some neurologic diseases or availability of facilities to appropriately diagnose and manage these patients. Equine neuroimaging is particularly challenging due to the large size of patients, configuration and weight limitations of CT and MR scanners, and issues associated with recovering a horse with neurologic problems from general anesthesia. Despite these limitations, advanced imaging techniques provide a great deal of useful information about the health status of the equine nervous system that is

The author has nothing to disclose.

Department of Clinical Sciences, College of Veterinary Medicine, Cornell University, C2 512 Veterinary Medical Center, Box 36, Ithaca, NY 14853, USA

E-mail address: pvs2@cornell.edu

vetequine.theclinics.com

important for making a diagnosis, planning treatment, or providing prognostic information to guide owner choices regarding decisions about patient care.

SELECTING AN IMAGING EXAMINATION

An imaging examination should be performed when there is a reasonable benefit to the patient that is justified for cost and risk, such as making a diagnosis, planning a surgery, or monitoring disease progression or treatment response. The impact of new neuroimaging technologies on improved patient care is undisputed. However, the exquisite depictions of anatomy and function generated by modern technology should not distract clinicians from the limitations and potential harms of radiologic diagnosis that always exist: the greatest patient risk is needless exposure to nonbeneficial downstream testing and inappropriate treatment related to misdiagnosis and overdiagnosis of common but unimportant findings.[2] Potential harms are mitigated by careful selection of the imaging examination, which includes examining the correct body region, using suitable imaging methods, and not performing unnecessary imaging. Obviously, the opportunity to make a diagnosis is missed when the correct body region is not examined or an unsuitable imaging method is used, and unnecessary imaging increases client cost and risk for misdiagnosis. Careful selection of the imaging examination is based on understanding the likelihood of disease and the accuracy of the various imaging methods.

Selection typically begins with neuroanatomic localization of the lesion to focus the imaging examination on a particular body region and thus avoid unnecessary imaging. Furthermore, neuroanatomic localization may limit the choice of available imaging modalities due to practical reasons. For example, horses with spinal disease may have a lesion localized to the cervical region (C1-C5), cervicothoracic region (C6-T2), thoracolumbar region (T3-L3), or lumbosacral region (L4-S5). Most CT scanners, however, cannot examine the vertebral column of adult horses caudal to the mid cervical region. Neuroanatomic localization often is made by physical examination, which occasionally is combined with a preliminary imaging examination to further localize a lesion to direct more exacting imaging methods. For treatment planning or monitoring the site of the lesion often is known beforehand, which facilitates selection of the examination. Next, selection is based on optimizing detection of the suspected lesion, which relies on having a prioritized list of differential diagnoses, an understanding of the types of lesions that may be produced by those diseases, and the accuracy of the different modalities to detect certain types of pathology. For example, if the disease is associated with acute hemorrhage, small calcifications, small accumulations of gas, or fine bone changes, then CT may be preferable due to high sensitivity for these conditions and high spatial resolution without superimposition of structures. If a seizure-related disorder such as hypoxic ischemic encephalopathy in neonatal foals or adult-onset idiopathic epilepsy is suspected, then MRI is preferable due to its high contrast resolution and sensitivity for soft tissue pathology.

In horses with neurologic disease, the neurocranium (brain and supporting structures) and cervical vertebral column (cervical spinal cord and supporting structures) are the most frequently examined body regions. Imaging of the thoracolumbar or lumbosacral vertebral column often is problematic due to patient size and inherent limitations of imaging equipment. Rarely, ultrasonography is used to evaluate peripheral nerves or other soft-tissue structures, or scintigraphy to identify elusive bone lesions. The most commonly used imaging techniques are radiography, myelography, CT, and MRI. Each of these modalities has advantages and disadvantages. Radiography generally is insensitive unless the disease is severe (**Fig. 1**).

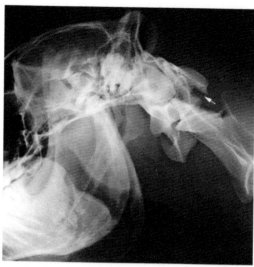

Fig. 1. Lateral radiograph of a 19-year-old Welsh stallion with tetraparesis due to an acute traumatic fracture of the atlas (*arrow*) with moderate displacement. Additionally, there is substantial hemorrhage into the guttural pouches with compression of the nasopharynx.

However, it is affordable, does not require general anesthesia, can be used to evaluate the entire head and neck, and can provide useful information. Cervical myelography is the only method available to routinely evaluate the caudal cervical spinal cord of adult horses. CT often can examine the entire head but only the cranial half of the neck (although that depends on the size of the horse and length of the neck). MRI generally can evaluate the head and maybe the first one or two cervical vertebrae of adult horses. In foals, more of the spine may be examined due to their smaller size. When cost, availability, patient risk, and size limitations are not factors, then cross-sectional imaging (CT/MRI) is preferred due to superior depiction of morphologic changes.

When comparing CT and MRI, it is commonly noted that MRI is good for soft tissue and CT is good for bone, but this notion is an oversimplification. For example, CT is excellent for examining the soft tissues of the thorax and abdomen, and MRI is excellent for detecting certain types of bone pathology. The difference between the two is that MRI has better contrast resolution and CT has better spatial resolution (compared to each other).[3] Improved contrast resolution is important for distinguishing between different soft tissues like white matter, gray matter, and CSF. Improved spatial resolution is better for examining fine anatomic features such as bone trabeculae. As such, MRI generally is preferred for examining the brain or spinal cord whenever reasonable. CT and MRI are both good for examining the supporting soft and hard tissues of the central nervous system, but they provide different information and the optimal examination varies with the type of disease. CT also may be preferable when a quick examination is desired, such as with acute trauma, or when computed reconstructions provide helpful depictions of the disease process (**Fig. 2**). Occasionally, both examinations together may provide a more complete picture of the pathology (**Fig. 3**). The art of medical imaging is obtaining useful lesion localization and contrast between tissues of interest, which is accomplished through choice of modality and proper setting of acquisition parameters.[3] Additionally, intravenous

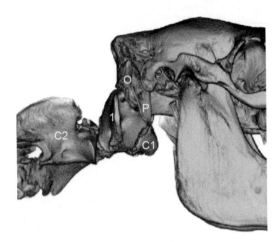

Fig. 2. Three-dimensional CT reconstruction (bone window) of a 4-month-old Friesian colt with occipitoatlantoaxial malformation, viewed from the horse's right. The atlas is attached to the squamous part of the occipital bone (O) and rotated approximately 90 degrees relative to the axis (C2): note that the wings of the atlas (1) are parallel to the paracondylar process (P) and the ventral arch of the atlas (C1) is immediately ventral to the paracondylar process.

contrast material may be used for both CT and MRI to improve lesion detection, better define altered morphology, and provide improve anatomic detail.

When selecting an imaging examination it is efficient to have established protocols for particular conditions: this is relatively easy to develop for common problems like cervical stenotic myelopathy (CSM) or temporohyoid osteoarthropathy (THO). Many other equine neurologic diseases are uncommon and occur sporadically. In these cases, flexibility is important and patient care may be optimized by tailoring the imaging examination to the particular needs of that patient based on the discussed principles.

ANATOMY

Anatomic knowledge is important for diagnosis, surgical planning, monitoring, and determining the clinical relevance of a lesion. If a neurologic lesion is clinically relevant, then its anatomic location should correspond to the observed clinical signs. For example, one might consider the laterality of the lesion and whether ipsilateral or contralateral clinical signs are expected. If a lesion is located in an area inconsistent with the clinical signs, then that lesion may be a diversion or associated with more extensive disease that is not easily detected by imaging (eg, elevated intracranial pressure). For intracranial lesions, an initial approach for anatomic localization during imaging is to first place the lesion in 1 of 6 major regions: (1) telencephalon (cerebrum), (2) diencephalon (thalamus, hypothalamus), (3) mesencephalon (mid-brain), (4) ventral metencephalon (pons), (5) dorsal metencephalon (cerebellum), or (6) myelenecephalon (medulla or medulla oblongata). Once a major region is identified, then anatomic references may be used to identify specific nuclei and tracts to relate to clinical signs. Note that there are differences between the anatomic regions that are defined by physical examination versus imaging (**Fig. 4**). During neurologic

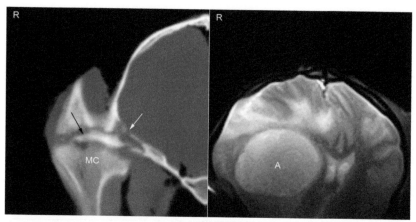

Fig. 3. Transverse CT scan (bone window) of the right temporomandibular joint (*left*) and transverse T2-weighted MRI of the brain (*right*) of a 2-year-old thoroughbred mare that sustained head trauma 4 weeks earlier. During physical examination, the horse was obtunded and blind in the left eye. A draining tract was present over the right temporomandibular joint. Postmortem CT scan discloses signs of infectious arthritis of the right temporomandibular joint with sequestrum (*black arrow*): note the irregular lysis on the articular surface of the mandibular condyle (MC). The infection continued into the cranial cavity (*white arrow*) and the right cerebral hemisphere contained a large intra-axial abscess (A) with cerebral edema and a midline shift to the left. R, right.

examination an intracranial lesion often is localized to 1 of 3 regions: (1) prosencephalon (forebrain), (2) caudal brainstem, or (3) cerebellum. The difference is that the forebrain is the combination of the cerebral hemispheres and diencephalon, and the caudal brainstem is the combination of the mesencephalon, ventral metencephalon and myelencephalon. Therefore, imaging usually provides a more specific description of the anatomic localization.

Another important anatomic relationship is between the foramina of the neurocranium and their associated soft-tissue structures. The neurocranium is the part of the skull that bounds the cranial cavity, which contains the brain, and is made up of the ethmoid, frontal, parietal, occipital, sphenoid, and temporal bones. The cranial cavity is divided into supratentorial and infratentorial parts by the tentorium osseum cerebelli. The neurocranium has a dorsal portion called the calvaria and a ventral portion called the base of the cranium, which contains many openings for nerves and blood vessels (**Table 1**).[4] During CT, the openings in the cranial base are identified to infer the location of the associated soft-tissue structures. During MRI, some individual nerves and blood vessels may be seen directly and more easily than the corresponding osseous opening. These openings (eg, fissure, foramina) may be viewed from the external or internal surfaces of the neurocranium. On the external surface, the openings on the caudomedial aspect of the orbit are ethmoidal foramen, optic canal, orbital fissure, trochlear foramen, rostral-alar foramen, unpaired alar foramen, and caudal-alar foramen (**Fig. 5A**). In the temporal region, there are retroarticular foramen, external acoustic meatus, and stylomastoid foramen (**Fig. 6**).[4] On the internal surface, the cranial base is divided from rostral to caudal into 3 shallow depressions called fossa. The rostral-cranial fossa extends from the cribiform plate to the orbitosphenoidal crest and contains the optic canal (**Fig. 5B**).[4] The middle-cranial fossa includes the hypophyseal fossa and piriform fossa and bilateral grooves extending to the

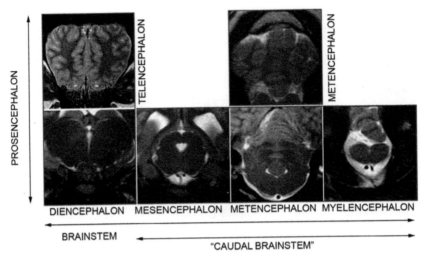

Fig. 4. T2-weighted, transverse, MRI of an adult horse's brain to depict various anatomic regions recognizable during imaging and the relationship with neuroanatomic localization during physical examination. During physical examination, an intracranial lesion may be localized to the prosencephalon, "caudal brainstem," or cerebellum. During imaging, an intracranial lesion may be localized more specifically. The anatomic level of the lesion is recognized by the cross-sectional silhouette of the cerebrum (telencephalon), the cerebellum (dorsal metencephalon), and the anatomic brain stem (diencephalon, mesencephalon, ventral metencephalon, and myelencephalon). The cross-sectional appearance of the ventricular system also is helpful for determining the level of a lesion.

orbital fissure, thorough which the optic, oculomotor, and trochlear nerves pass.[4] The openings found are orbital fissure, round foramen, and trochlear foramen (see **Fig. 5**B).[4] The caudal-cranial fossa extends caudal from the middle-cranial fossa to the foramen magnum and contains: foramen lacerum, jugular foramen, and hypoglossal canal (**Fig. 7**).[4] Also on the interior surface, in the temporal region dorsolateral to the caudal cranial fossa, is the internal acoustic meatus (see **Fig. 7**A).[4]

INTRODUCTORY CROSS-SECTIONAL (CT/MRI) INTERPRETATION PRINCIPLES

This section reviews introductory interpretation principles that are necessary to begin systematic evaluation of the neuroimaging examination. In practice many more imaging signs are used: also, certain patterns of signs are associated with particular diseases.

Interpretation begins by systematically evaluating the images for abnormalities. Abnormalities or lesions are recognized when there is either (1) a change in morphology or (2) a change in signal intensity (SI) during MRI or attenuation (density) during CT. If a disease does not produce a change in morphology, SI, or attenuation, then the results of the examination are apt to be negative for that disease. Alterations of SI or attenuation indicate abnormal changes in tissues, which is why they are so helpful to recognize pathology. By convention, if a tissue has a higher SI or attenuation, then that tissue is depicted as whiter; lower SI or attenuation as blacker. Explicit changes to a tissue's SI or attenuation may be characteristic of certain diseases or processes. For example, during CT, a hyperattenuating intracranial lesion indicates more dense structures such as calcification, iodinated contrast medium,

Table 1
Comparison between openings of the cranium and transmitted structures

ID	Osseous Opening	Soft-Tissue Contents
a	Cribiform plate	CN I—Olfactory nerve
b	Optic canal	CN II—Optic nerve
c	Orbital fissure	CN III—Oculomotor nerve CN V$_1$—Ophthalmic nerve CN VI—Abducent nerve External ophthalmic vein
d	Trochlear foramen	CN IV—Trochlear nerve
e	Ethmoidal foramen	CN V$_1$—(Ophthalmic nerve) Ethmoidal nerve
f	Round foramen	CN V$_2$—Maxillary nerve
g	Rostral-alar foramen	CN V$_2$—Maxillary nerve Maxillary artery
h	Caudal-alar foramen	Maxillary artery
i	Unpaired-alar foramen	Rostral-deep-temporal artery
j	Retroarticular foramen	Emissary veins for the temporal sinus
k	Internal acoustic meatus	CN VII—Facial nerve CN VIII—Vestibulocochlear nerve
l	Stylomastoid foramen	CN VII—Facial nerve
m	External acoustic meatus	
n	Foramen lacerum (oval notch)	CN V$_3$—Mandibular nerve
o	Foramen lacerum (carotid notch)	Internal carotid artery
p	Foramen lacerum (spinous notch)	Middle-meningeal artery
q	Jugular foramen	CN IX—Glossopharyngeal nerve CN X—Vagus nerve CN XI—Accessory nerve
r	Hypoglossal foramen	CN XII—Hypoglossal nerve Condylar artery and vein

Abbreviation: CN V, trigeminal nerve.
Nerves shown in parentheses give rise to the indicated nerve.

acute hemorrhage, or certain tumors. A hypoattenuating lesion may indicate edema, brain atrophy with volume replacement by CSF, or certain artifacts. In MRI the situation is more complicated because multiple tissue characteristics (eg, T1, T2, diffusion) may be evaluated. Furthermore, special sequences may be used to null (make dark) the SI from fat or CSF so that high SI lesions stand out from fat or CSF. The key to recognizing certain diseases is by recognizing the pattern of altered tissue characteristics. Therefore, neuroimaging interpretation is dependent on familiarity with normal morphology and normal tissue characteristics as depicted by the different imaging methods, as well as what specific changes might indicate.

Once a lesion is identified because of altered morphology, SI, or attenuation, then the next most useful clue for making a diagnosis is the anatomic location of the lesion. It may be prosaic but a lesion confined to the ependyma is likely an ependymal disease such as ependymitis; a lesion associated with the meninges is likely meningitis or meningioma. Therefore, accurate identification of the abnormal tissue or precise location of a lesion is extremely important because certain diseases occur in precise anatomic locations. Subsequently, additional imaging signs are used to

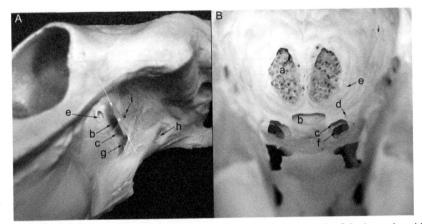

Fig. 5. Equine skull: (*A*) lateral view of the left orbit (rostral is to the left of the image) and (*B*) caudodorsal-oblique view of the rostral and middle fossae (calvaria removed; rostral is at the top of the image). The white arrows indicate the petrosal crest: deep to this structure lies the trochlear foramen (*). See **Table 1** for legend.

further refine the differential diagnosis. For example, if the meningeal lesion is a focal mass, then meningioma is prioritized. If the meninges are locally extensive or diffusely thick, then meningitis is prioritized (**Fig. 8**). Some additional anatomic distinctions that are important are whether lesions are predominantly confined to white matter, grey matter, ventricles, central canal, choroid plexus (**Fig. 9**), pituitary gland (eg, pituitary macroadenoma), or a combination of tissues. Other diseases—such as trauma, abscess, some inflammatory diseases, neoplasia, vascular occlusive disease—affect the central nervous system (CNS) at random or unpredictable locations. Systemic, toxic, or metabolic diseases frequently produce a bilateral, anatomic-symmetric distribution of lesions because the whole brain is exposed to the insult, but only

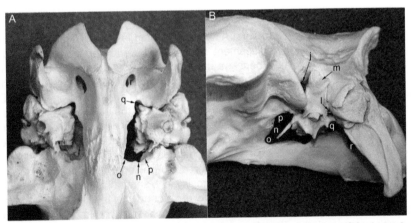

Fig. 6. Equine skull: (*A*) ventral view of the skull base (caudal is at the top of the image) and (*B*) lateral view of the left side of the caudal skull (caudal is at the right of the image). See **Table 1** for legend.

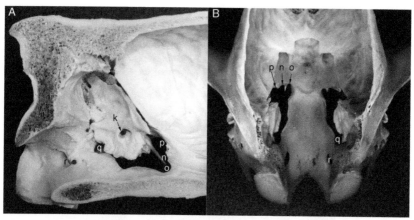

Fig. 7. . Equine skull: (*A*) medial view of the caudal skull (caudal is at the left of the image) and (*B*) dorsal view of the caudal fossa (calvaria removed; rostral is at the top of the image). See **Table 1** for legend.

certain nuclei or tracts may be susceptible to injury (eg, nigropallidal encephaloma-lacia).[5] The term "bilateral, anatomic-symmetric" indicates a distribution that affects the nuclei and tracts on both the left and right sides—not that the left and right lesions look identical.

Another helpful approach for characterizing abnormalities is to determine whether a lesion is intra-axial or extra-axial. Axis determination is important because it divides diseases into two large groups: those arising from inside or outside of the CNS. An intra-axial lesion is one that arises from within the parenchyma of the brain or spinal cord (eg, gliomas). An extra-axial lesion is one that arises from the meninges, subarachnoid space, subdural space, epidural space (**Fig. 10**), cranium, vertebra, or

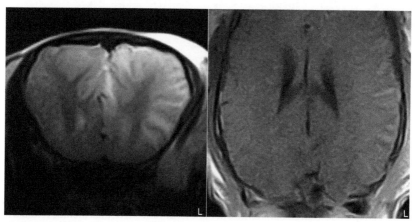

Fig. 8. T2-weighted, transverse MRI and a T1-weighted, dorsal MRI following intravenous administration of contrast material in a 6-week-old thoroughbred colt with seizures due to meningitis. Note that the meninges in the left cerebral hemisphere have higher signal intensity on both scans: they are seen as they extend deep into the sulci.

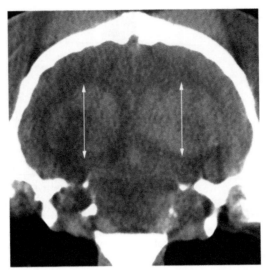

Fig. 9. Transverse, CT scan (soft-tissue window) of a 7.5-year-old shire mare with depression, obtundation, cortical vision loss (left-sided), and fever associated with 2 large, heterogeneously, hyperdense cholseterinic granulomas filling the lateral ventricles and compressing the adjacent cerebrum.

other supporting soft tissue. Lesions that originate far outside of the neurocranium or vertebral column but are extensive enough to involve the CNS also are extra-axial (**Fig. 11**). For spinal lesions, an intra-axial lesion commonly is described as intramedullary, and an extra-axial lesion as either intradural-extramedullary or extradural. An

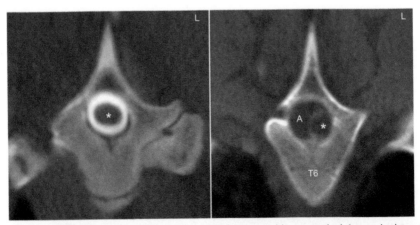

Fig. 10. Transverse CT myelograms (bone window) of a 9-year-old, castrated miniature donkey with pelvic limb paralysis due to an epidural abscess at the level of T6. (*Left*) Normal thoracic vertebra from the same patient: note the size and attenuation of the ring of contrast material that surrounds the spinal cord (*). At T6 the ring of contrast medium surrounding the spinal cord (*) is severely attenuated, small, distorted, and displaced to the left. In the right side of the vertebral canal, the abscess (*A*) is seen as a homogeneous soft-tissue density with poorly defined borders.

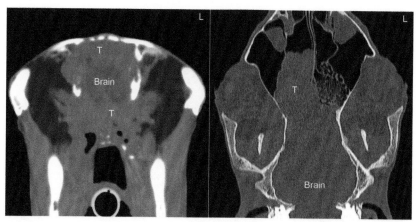

Fig. 11. Transverse CT scan (soft-tissue window) (*left*) and dorsal CT scan (bone window) (*right*) of a 10-year-old appendix horse gelding with facial swelling, nasal discharge, depression, and blindness due to a locally extensive nasal adenocarcinoma (T) that extends into the cranial cavity. L = left.

intra-axial lesion may be recognized when it is surrounded by normal brain or spinal cord on every image: if an intra-axial lesion contacts the surface and is not completely surrounded by the CNS, then it often has a narrow base of surface contact. In contrast, broad-based surface contact is characteristic of an extra-axial lesion. It is not always possible to distinguish whether a lesion is intra-axial or extra-axial—especially when a lesion is very large, originates near the surface of the CNS, or originates from an extra-axial tissue that is normally surrounded by CNS (eg, falx cerebri).

CERVICAL STENOTIC MYELOPATHY

CSM is known by a variety of names (eg, "Wobbler's syndrome," cervical vertebral malformation malarticulation, cervical vertebral instability) and is a multifactorial disease characterized by diffuse malformation and malarticulation of the cervical vertebrae with static or dynamic stenosis of the vertebral canal causing one or more sites of spinal cord compression. Stenosis may be due to a bone malformation, an abnormal soft tissue structure (eg, ligamentous or joint capsule hypertrophy, synovial cysts), and/or instability of the vertebral column. In older horses, spinal cord compression typically occurs in the caudal neck and is associated with osteoarthrosis of the synovial joints. In younger horses, spinal cord compression tends toward the mid neck but any site may be affected.

Radiography may be performed initially to rule out other causes, such as trauma, and provide supportive evidence of CSM. Cervical myelography often is performed after excluding other diagnoses, such as equine protozoal myelitis, to further reduce diagnostic uncertainty, to assess disease severity, or to plan surgery. Unfortunately, both imaging examinations do not consistently specify the actual cause of compression (eg, synovial cyst, ligamentous hypertrophy, instability, bone malformation), which might direct different types of treatment or prognosis. Additionally, false-positive and false-negative results are possible.[6] As such, the final clinical diagnosis is based on a combination of findings that include imaging. The insensitivity of these imaging methods to consistently detect compression may be explained in part by the

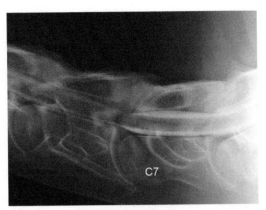

Fig. 12. Lateral myelogram of the caudal neck in a 2-year-old foreign warm blood gelding with progressive ataxia with two week rapid progression due to an epidural hematoma at C6-C7. Note that columns of contrast material are thin and displaced ventrally (especially the dorsal column) at C6-C7. No bone malformation is detected.

source of compression, which is commonly located dorsolaterally.[7] Typical radiographic projections (lateral and ventrodorsal) are not optimal for depicting this type of compression unless it is severe: oblique projections may be more informative.[7] Additionally, static radiographs may not disclose the dynamic nature of the compression: obtaining myelograms with neck in flexed, neutral, and extended positions is one way to address this concern. For many years, a simple metric was sought to accurately distinguish horses with CSM; recently, intervertebral and intravertebral ratios were shown to be unreliable as interobserver and intraobserver measurements varied 5% to 10%.[8] Probably the best approach to radiography and myelography interpretation is visual inspection of the images by experienced readers. CSM is more apt to be correctly diagnosed when the lesions are severe or more signs of CSM are detected (eg, reduced minimum height of the vertebral canal, reduced minimum height of the columns of contrast material, excessive length of the lamina caudally, dorsal flaring of the caudal epiphysis, abnormal alignment, or subluxation of the vertebral column).[9]

Other diseases may result in a compressive myelopathy but are distinguished from CSM (eg, epidural abscess, neoplasm, trauma, congenital vertebral malformation, intervertebral disk herniation, epidural hematoma). Epidural hematomas tend to occur in the caudal cervical region, might have a history of trauma, and may produce neck pain and tetraparesis of equal severity in all 4 limbs.[10] Epidural hematomas may mimic CSM and should be considered in the differential diagnosis for an extradural spinal cord compression, especially when no other sign of CSM is present (**Fig. 12**).

TEMPOROHYOID OSTEOARTHROPATHY

THO is a disease characterized by progressive bone proliferation of the temporohyoid joint and hyoid apparatus due to unknown reasons: some proposed causes are infection of the upper respiratory tract or ear, previous trauma, or progressive degenerative joint disease (**Fig. 13**). A variety of clinical signs may be observed including head shaking, facial and/or vestibulocochlear nerve deficits, painful or difficult eating, and rarely seizures.[11] Diagnosis frequently is made using endoscopy and skull radiography, but these examinations have limitations.[11] CT allows for

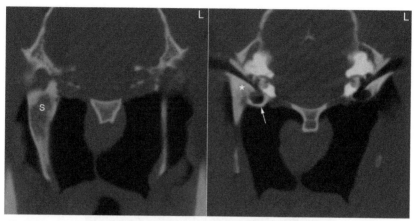

Fig. 13. Transverse CT scans (bone window) of the temporal region of a 16-year-old quarter horse gelding with ataxia and left temporohyoid osteoarthropaty. (*Left*) Thick right stylohyoid bone (S) that is fused to the temporal bone (*). (*Right*) Increased thickness of the right tympanic bulla (*arrow*) and mild fluid within the right tympanic cavity. L = left.

evaluation of the entire hyoid apparatus and the left and right temporal regions without superimposition of structures. CT also is more sensitive to detecting increased thickness of the hyoid bones, ankylosis, temporal bone fracture, and bilateral disease even when clinical signs suggest a unilateral problem.[11] In horses with a temporal bone fracture, THO is a common coexisting finding.[12] However, most horses with THO do not have a temporal bone fracture.[12] Temporal bone fractures do not denote whether facial and/or vestibulocochlear nerve deficits are present, and clinical findings of facial and/or vestibulocochlear nerve deficits do not specify whether the temporal bone is fractured (**Fig. 14**).[12]

SUMMARY

Neuroimaging underwent a dramatic revolution during the past few decades due to the development of new technologies that produce exquisite images of patient morphology and function, new technologies that store and distribute information more efficiently, and research that has improved understanding of pathogenesis and effective clinical use of new imaging methods. Advanced equine neuroimaging is a specialized field with unique challenges associated with patient size, availability of equipment, using equipment designed for humans, small sample size for various diseases, and issues associated with recovering a horse with neurologic problems from general anesthesia. Despite these challenges, modern imaging techniques provide much useful information in horses with neurologic disease that are important for making a diagnosis, planning treatment, monitoring patient response, or providing prognostic information to guide owner choices regarding decisions about patient care. In particular, CT and MRI have been beneficial in diagnosing several equine neurologic diseases including congenital malformations (eg, hydrocephalus), equine protozoal myeloencephalitis, strangles (*Streptococcus equi* ssp. *equi*) abscesses, nigropallidal encephalomalacia,[5] pituitary macroadenomas, cholesterinic granulomas, THO, CSM, trauma, and various neoplasms. Optimizing equine neuroimaging starts with selecting an appropriate examination, understanding the prior probability of disease and the capabilities of the different imaging technologies, understanding

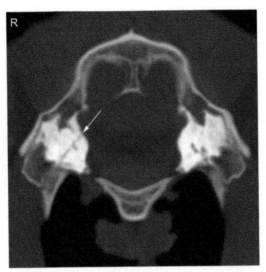

Fig. 14. Transverse CT scan (bone window) of a 3-year-old Appaloosa stallion with a right head tilt, neck swelling, and ataxia after being found cast in a stall 10 days earlier. Note the dorsomedial-ventrolateral fracture of the petrosal pyramid of the right-temporal bone (*arrow*). R, right.

normal anatomy and pathogenesis, and having a systematic approach to review the images. Advanced equine neuroimaging will continue to evolve as more of the challenges are overcome and new research is produced on the effective use of imaging methods and understanding of specific diseases.

REFERENCES

1. Chong BW, Sanders JA, Jones GM. Functional magnetic resonance imaging. In: Orrison WW, editor. Neuroimaging. Philadelphia: WB Saunders; 2000. p. 60–85.
2. Hillman BJ, Goldsmith JC. The uncritical use of high-tech medical imaging. N Engl J Med 2010;363(1)1:4-6.3.
3. Sanders JA. Computed tomography and magnetic resonance imaging. In: Orrison WW. Neuroimaging, W.B. Saunders Company, Philadelphia;2000:12-36.4.
4. König HE, Leibich HG. Veterinary anatomy of domestic mammals. Textbook and colour atlas, 3rd ed. Stuttgart, Germany: Schattauer GmbH;2005:3070.
5. Sanders SG, Tucker RL, Bagley RS, Gavin PR. Magnetic resonance imaging features of equine nigropallidal encephalomalacia. Vet Radiol Ultrasound 2001;42(4):291–6.
6. Van Biervliet J, Scrivani PV, Divers T, Erb HN, deLahunta A, Nixon A. Evaluation of decision criteria for detection of spinal cord compression based on cervical myelography in horses: 38 cases (1981-2001). Equine Vet J 2004;36(1):14–20.
7. Claridge HAH, Piercy RJ, Parry A, Weller R. The 3D anatomy of the cervical articular process joints in the horse and their topographical relationship to the spinal cord. Equine Vet J 2010;42(8):726–31.
8. Scrivani PV, Levine JM, Holmes NL, Furr M, Divers TJ, Cohen HD. Observer agreement study of cervical-vertebral ratios in horses. Accepted, Equine Vet J 2010; DOI: 10.1111/j.2042-3306.2010.00300.x.

9. Hudson NPH, Mayhew IG. Radiographic and myelographic assessment of the equine cervical vertebral column and spinal cord. Equine Veterinary Education 2005;17(1): 34–8.

10. Gold JR, Divers TJ, Miller AJ, Scrivani PV, Perkins GA, Van Biervliet J, deLahunta A. Cervical vertebral spinal hematomas in 4 horses. J Vet Intern Med 2008;22(2): 481–5.

11. Hilton H, Puchalski SM, Aleman M. The computed tomographic appearance of equine temporohyoid osteoarthropathy. Vet Radiol Ultrasound 2009;50(2):151–6.

12. Pownder SL, Scrivani PV, Bezuidenhout A, Divers DJ, Ducharme NG. Computed tomography of temporal bone fractures and temporal region anatomy in horses. J Vet Intern Med 2010;24:398–406.

Neuro-ophthalmology in Horses

Nita L. Irby, DVM

KEYWORDS

- Equine • Split lid tarsorrhaphy • Eye • Neurology
- Neuro-ophthalmology • Horse

THE NEURO-OPHTHALMOLOGIC EXAMINATION

A complete neuro-ophthalmologic assessment is part of every ophthalmic and neurologic examination. Cranial nerves II, III, IV, V, VI, VII, and VIII and a portion of the sympathetic and parasympathetic innervation to the head can be evaluated on or near the eye by general observation, by vision assessment, by assessing the menace response, ocular reflexes (pupillary light, dazzle, and palpebral), and by observing globe and lid movement, positions and response to touch. Neuro-ophthalmic assessment of the equine patient begins with a routine general history that should also include questions related to use of the horse, performance, and visual acuity in bright and dim light situations. The neuro-ophthalmic examination should be performed, whenever possible, in a well-lit environment that can be darkened completely as required. Some patients require sedation before any portion of an ophthalmic examination can proceed but ideally the examination is completed without sedation and without the use of any topical or local anesthetic agents. Equipment needs are minimal: a focal halogen or other bright light source such as a Finhoff transilluminator or otoscope light (nonmagnified) and a towel to use, if needed, as a blindfold. The clinician is cautioned to *never* use an LED penlight or other LED light source unless its brightness has been previously assessed on a human, as some LED penlights are sufficiently bright as to create discomfort similar to that of looking at the sun and leave a retinal afterimage that may persist more than 24 hours.

General observations are important before examining the eyes and head more closely. Note the head and neck carriage and symmetry of the structures of the head and face with particular attention to the movement and position of the ears, nostrils, eyelids, and globes. Note any deviation of the nose and any swelling evident or palpable in the cheek pouches, all of which may indicate facial nerve dysfunction. Note any head or neck sweating as well as any other hair coat, muscular, or obvious bony abnormalities. Assess the relative position of the globes in the orbit (enophthalmos,

The author has nothing to disclose.

Department of Clinical Sciences, Cornell University College of Veterinary Medicine, Room C2 534, Ithaca, NY 14853, USA

E-mail address: nli2@cornell.edu

Vet Clin Equine 27 (2011) 455–479
doi:10.1016/j.cveq.2011.08.010
0749-0739/11/$ – see front matter © 2011 Elsevier Inc. All rights reserved.

Box 1
Conditions causing ptosis in the horse

1. Ocular pain or discomfort due to any cause (ulcers, foreign bodies, uveitis)—squinting due to pain may mimic ptosis

2. Enophthalmos due to any cause

3. Facial paralysis (ptosis usually marked due to loss of angularis oculi medialis function, lid tone reduced due to loss of tone in orbicularis oculi)

4. Loss of sympathetic innervation: Horner's syndrome (mild ptosis, dropped eyelash angle in affected eye); grass sickness (bilaterally dropped eyelashes; lid tone usually normal)—loss of tone and function of Mueller's muscle

5. Oculomotor nerve dysfunction (mild ptosis, lid tone usually good)—loss of levator papebrae function

6. Botulism—decreased lid tone is one of the hallmarks of the disease, may be accompanied by mild mydriasis in foals

---

exophthalmos) and obvious altered size of either globe (buphthalmos, phthisis bulbi, microphthalmos, etc.), and take note of the patient's behavior and awareness of its environment. Check for ptosis (see **Box 1**). Check for voluntary movements of the eyelids (normal blinking - see **Box 2**) and the frequency, symmetry, and completeness of normal blinking (a normal horse at rest blinks approximately 15 ± 10 times per minute; the right and left eye can blink asynchronously and incomplete blinks occur approximately one-third of the time; blinks accompanied by globe retraction are rare unless facial paralysis or irritation such as an eyelid foreign body is present). Approaching the patient more closely, note the amount and character of any ocular discharge. While at a safe distance in front of the patient note the shape and size of the palpebral fissures and, looking squarely at the face, compare the angle of the upper eyelashes bilaterally, which in a normal horse should be approximately perpendicular to the face or angled slightly down no more than 10 to 15 degrees (lashes that point or droop more ventrally may indicate loss of sympathetic tone to the lid or, more commonly, may indicate eye pain, wherein the accompanying blepharospasm, enophthalmos, ptosis, or possible swelling may direct the lashes downward) (**Figs. 1** and **2**). Note the presence of "bags" under either or both eyes that often accompany eye inflammation or orbit edema in the equine patient (see **Fig. 2**). The facial fold immediately dorsal to the lashes, known as the supraciliary sulcus, and the sulcus immediately ventral to the orbit rim should be assessed bilaterally for

---

Box 2
Muscles and nerves involved in closing the equine upper eyelid

Orbicularis oculi	Facial (VII)
Muscle	Innervation
Levator palpebrae superioris	Oculomotor (III)
Levator angularis oculi medialis	Facial (VII)
Orbitalis (Mueller's muscle)	Sympathetic LMN
Arectores ciliorum (contraction maintains eyelashes erect)	Sympathetic LMN

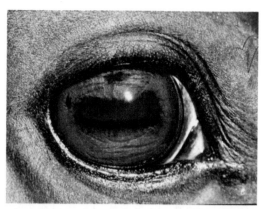

Fig. 1. A normal equine right eye (11-year-old thoroughbred). Note the size, shape, and position of the normal pupil in bright light and the relationship of the globe to the eyelids, as well as the membrana nictitans. The eyelashes or cilia on the upper lid are in normal position, perpendicular to the head (and, as a result, are hard to see in the picture). There are several creases present nasally in the upper lid that dorsally become the supraciliary sulcus, a good place to look to assess subtle orbit or globe swelling. Also note that the eyelid is open to a slightly greater degree at the junction between the medial third and lateral two-thirds of the lid, the location of the insertion of the *levator angularis oculi medialis,* which is innervated by cranial nerve VII.

symmetry (subtle enophthlamos often causes slight deepening of this sulcus and buphthalmos or exophthalmos will cause the sulcus to be shallow or absent) (see **Figs. 1 and 2**). Retropulsion of each globe should be performed at this time to assess the nictitating membrane, its normal excursion, and, indirectly, the orbit contents. Note the size, clarity, shape, and contour of each cornea and its position in relation to the lid margins and the orbit bones (see **Fig. 1**). Note the amount of conjunctiva exposed in each eye (careful observation may be required if the perilimbal conjunctiva

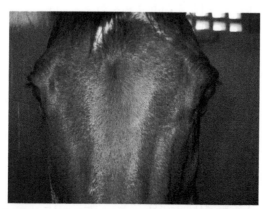

Fig. 2. Mild exophthalmos, subtle filling of the supraciliary and orbital sulci and slight lower lid edema in this horse's blind left eye. Retropulsion of the left eye was slightly reduced. Eyelash position is normal. A sinoethmoid neoplasia was diagnosed on CT. The horse was euthanized at home 3.5 years later when behavior changes developed.

Table 1
Cranial nerves examined during routine eye examinations

Nerve	Name	Clinical Function	Assessment
II	Optic	Afferent pathway for light and vision; sensory input contributes to pupil responses and development of conjugate eye movements	History; vision assessment; menace response (II → VII), pupillary light reflex (II → III), dazzle reflex (II → VII)
III	Oculomotor	Motor to the dorsal, medial, and ventral rectus and ventral oblique muscles of the globe and motor to the levator palpebrae superioris of upper lid; autonomic (parasympathetic) motor to the sphincter muscle of the pupil	Move head medially and laterally. If the globe adducts (moves medially) then the medial rectus is functioning (DR and VR function are harder to assess); check for ptosis (Box 2); check pupillary light reflex observing for pupil constriction
IV	Trochlear	Motor to the dorsal oblique muscle	Observation of pupil orientation (with trochlear paralysis the medial portion of the pupil is directed dorsally causing an "up-and-in" gaze)
V	Trigeminal	Sensory to the face; motor to the muscles of mastication	Palpebral reflex assessment at the medial canthus (ophthalmic branch of V) and lateral canthus (maxillary branch of V); check sensation on chin (sensory part of mandibular branch); observe chewing, and palpate tone in temporal and masseter muscles (motor component of mandibular V); observe mandible position (may deviate slightly to normal side)[1p139]
VI	Abducent or abducens*	Motor to the lateral rectus and retractor bulbi muscles	Move head medially and laterally. If the eyes abduct (move laterally), the lateral rectus muscles are functional. Touch response: watch for globe retraction to corneal touch- not routinely recommended

| VII | Facial | Motor to muscles of facial expression (ears, eyelids, nose, cheeks) including the orbicularis oculi muscle and levator anguli oculi medialis. VII also carries from the brainstem to the petrous temporal bone the parasympathetic fibers to the lacrimal glands | Observe patient for facial symmetry, ear and nose position and movement (including nostrils) and absence of food boluses in cheeks; check palpebral reflex; assess eyelid tone; perform Schirmer tear test |
| VIII | Vestibular portion of the vestibulocochlear nerve | Integrates eye movements with head and body positions via the vestibular system | Observe the patient's eyes as you move the head side-to-side and up-and-down observing for normal and abnormal nystagmus |

* *Note.* Damage to one abducens nucleus, in contrast to a peripheral VI nerve lesion, results in a palsy of horizontal gaze in *both* eyes because of interneurons between the abducens nucleus and the contralateral oculomotor nucleus. The interneuron connection ensures congruity of movements of both eyes so that when one moves medially the other moves laterally.

Table 2
Neuro-ophthalmologic assessment summary

Lesion (all lesions on right side)	Menace Response	Pupil OS	Pupil OD	Palpebral Reflex OS	Palpebral Reflex OD	Upper Lid Position	Globe Position and Movement
OD Retina or optic nerve (severe)*	OS + OD –	Normal size Light in OS → OU constrict	Normal to slight ↑ size; Light in OD → No constriction OU (Note: cover OS and OD dilates immediately)	+	+	Normal OU	Normal OU
OD Retrobulbar, intraperiorbital lesion affecting II and III (parasympathetic III fibers only)	OS + OD –	Normal size Light in OS → only OS constricts	Widely dilated Light in OD → No constriction OU	+	+	Normal OU	Normal OU
OD Complete oculomotor nerve (III) lesion	OD + OD +	Normal size Light in OS → only OS constricts	Widely dilated Light in OD → only OS constricts	+	+	Slight ptosis OD (due to loss of innervation to the levator palpebrae superioris)	Ventrolateral strabismus that is present in all head positions; globe will not adduct when assessing normal nystagmus
OD Parasympathetic fibers of oculomotor nerve (III)	OS + OD +	Normal size Light in OS → only OS constricts	Widely dilated Light in OD → only OS constricts	+	+	Normal OU	Normal OU

OD Trochlear nerve (IV) lesion	OS + OD +	Normal size Light in OS → OU constrict	Normal size Light in OD OS → OU constrict See note† below: If lesion is peripheral trochlear nerve OD then the medial aspect of OD pupil will be rotated dorsally or exotorted (ie, the OD is counter clockwise rotated)†	+	+	Normal OU	Normal OU
OD Ophthalmic branch of V lesion	OS + OD +	Normal size Light in OS → OU constrict	Normal size; Light in OD → OU constrict	+	– when medial upper lid is touched; + when lower lid is touched laterally; – response when nasal septum is touched	Normal OU	Normal OU
OD Maxillary branch of V lesion	OS + OD +	Normal size Light in OS → OU constrict	Normal size Light in OD OS → OU constrict	+	+ when medial upper lid is touched; – when lower lid is touched laterally; + response when nasal septum is touched	Normal OU	Normal OU

(continued on next page)

Table 2
(continued)

Lesion (all lesions on right side)	Menace Response	Pupil OS	Pupil OD	Palpebral Reflex OS	Palpebral Reflex OD	Upper Lid Position	Globe Position and Movement
OD Mandibular branch of V lesion	OS + OD +	Normal size Light in OS → OU constrict	Normal size Light in OS → OU constrict	+	Right side masseter and temporal muscles ↓ tone or atrophic; jaw may deviate slightly to the left side; no sensation lower lip	Normal OU	Normal OU
OD Abducent nerve paralysis (VI)	OS + OD +	Normal size Light in OS → OU constrict	Normal size Light in OS → OU constrict	+	+	+	Inability to abduct the OD globe and medial strabismus; inability to retract the globe (unreliable to assess)
OD Facial paralysis (entire right side VII lesion)	OS + OD –	Normal size Light in OS → OU constrict	Normal size; Light in OD → OU constrict	+	–	Ptosis OD due to paralysis of levator anguli oculi muscle; no voluntary blinking OD; eyelashes dropped OD (ipsilateral ear droop; nose deviated to normal side)	Normal OU

| OD Sympathetic pathway lesion (OD Horner syndrome)‡ | OS + OD + | Normal size Light in OS → OU constrict | Slight miosis (which becomes more obvious when ambient lighting is dimmed) Light in OD → OU constrict | + | + | Slight ptosis; significantly dropped eyelash angle due to loss of innervation to the arrector ciliorum muscles) | Very slight enophthalmos and very slight nictitans elevation |

Modified from DeLahunta A, Glass E. Visual system. In: Veterinary Anatomy and Clinical Neurology. 3rd ed. St Louis: Saunders Elsevier, with permission.
This table assumes that there is no ocular pathology preventing pupil movement, function, and position in either eye such as synechiae, uveitis, iris atrophy, glaucoma, or previous drug administration (atropine, for example).
* PLR may persist even in advanced stages of some retinal diseases.
† *Note.* The trochlear nucleus is on the opposite side of the brain from the nerve termination. Therefore a lesion affecting the right trochlear nucleus will manifest as a left trochlear paralysis whereas a lesion affecting the nerve fibers beyond the rostral colliculus affects the ipsilateral eye.
‡ See text for lesion localization and additional discussion.

> **Box 3**
> **Notes on the neuro-ophthalmologic examination of foals**
>
> 1. The blinking component of the menace response is unreliable for 1 to 3 weeks or more (a normal, visual foal may not menace and the menace may be inconsistent between two eyes, possibly due to cerebellar immaturity).[3] Some foals will move away or startle in response to a confrontational, menacing gesture.
>
> 2. The pupillary light reflex may be slightly slower than an adult and the foal's pupil is notably rounder than the adult pupil.
>
> 3. Corneal sensation and tear production may be diminished in foals, especially in sick and neurologically abnormal foals. *All sick foals should be assessed daily for corneal ulcers* and the eyes treated as needed. Ocular surface lubrication four or more times a day should be provided to prevent ulcer formation.
>
> 4. A slight ventromedial or rotational strabismus may be seen in some foals less than 1 month of age (the nasal portion of the pupil is ventral to the lateral pupil). This is exaggerated in certain head positions.

is heavily pigmented) and assess the resting position of each membrana nictitans (third eyelid) for symmetry.

While still positioned safely in front of the patient, the examiner should hold a bright light near his or her own eyes but directed into the patient's eyes, to assess simultaneously the size and symmetry of each pupil. Pupils, having been observed in room light, should be assessed again in darkness after a few minutes of dark adaptation. Approaching the patient more closely, a general inspection of the each eye should be done next to ensure that further eye and eyelid manipulations will cause no harm. The orbit rim, periorbital bones, and zygomatic arch should be gently palpated, the patient's external lids inspected, and, once the integrity of the globe is confirmed normal, the exam can proceed. If a complete ophthalmic examination is being performed in conjunction with a neuro-ophthalmic exam, a Schirmer I tear test should be performed at this time in order to avoid stimulation of tear production. A Schirmer I tear test should be performed in every case of facial nerve (VII) paresis or paralysis as reduced tear production will occur if parasympathetic innervation to the lacrimal glands has been lost (parasympathetics to the lacrimal gland travel with cranial nerve VII). Cultures, if indicated, should be obtained at this time. The cranial nerve portion of the eye examination is completed next (tests performed and a simplified version of their corresponding nerve pathways are summarized in **Tables 1 and 2, Box 1**). Comments on the neuro-ophthalmologic examination of foals can be found in **Box 3**.

PALPEBRAL OR BLINK REFLEX (A V → VII REFLEX)

After the patient's voluntary blinking frequency and pattern are observed, a palpebral reflex should be elicited by gently tapping the upper and lower lids at the medial and lateral commissures of each eye; the patient should close the eyelids completely with each touch (in the equine patient, the upper lid excursion is normally much greater than that of the lower lid). When touching the medial upper lid, the examiner is assessing the ophthalmic branch of the trigeminal nerve (V_1) and when the lower lid is touched at the lateral canthus the maxillary branch of the trigeminal nerve (V_2) is stimulated. The efferent or motor portion of the reflex is carried in axons of the facial nerve (VII) to the orbicularis oculi muscle and when the orbicularis oculi muscle contracts the palpebral fissure closes. If there is no response when the medial canthus is stimulated the examiner should next gently touch the ipsilateral mucosa of the nasal septum, which is innervated by the same nerve, V_1, which innervates the medial canthus and cornea. If there is no response when the lateral canthus is stimulated the examiner should assess sensation over the maxillary portion of the face, the nostrils and the upper lip to further assess V_2. If the reflex is still questionable, the menace response will help to further assess facial nerve function.

MENACE RESPONSE TEST (A II → VII RESPONSE)

The "menace" is not a reflex but is a complicated, learned response that requires an intact visual pathway from the eye to the contralateral cerebral cortex then back to the eyelids via the ipsilateral facial nucleus in the brainstem. The response is rarely present in newborn foals but develops by 2 to 4 weeks of age. To perform the test, a quick, threatening, but nontactile gesture is directed toward one eye, ensuring that the gesticulation does not touch the cilia or sensory vibrissae near the eye or create an air current, all of which stimulate the corneal or palpebral reflexes (V → VII reflexes rather than the II → VII reflex desired). A positive response consists of ipsilateral eyelid closure, with or without retraction of the globe. Some patients may move their entire head away while others may startle (caution should be used performing the test in the nervous patient). The menace test should be repeated several times in all visual fields (nasal, temporal, dorsal, ventral, and axial). Gentle tapping of the face may be required to elicit the response initially and this may need to be repeated as testing proceeds if the patient becomes conditioned to the threatening gestures. Patients who fail to respond to menacing gestures should have optic nerve function (II) assessed via a pupillary light reflex assessment and facial nerve (VII) function assessed via palpebral reflex testing to ensure that they can blink. If the menace response is abnormal, the patient should be assessed for lesions in the retina, optic nerve, optic chiasm, and visual cortex. Diffuse cerebellar disease, usually an obvious clinical diagnosis, can cause bilaterally altered or absent menace responses in the presence of normal vision, pupillary light reflex, and palpebral reflexes[1(p400)] or menace responses may be absent ipsilateral to focal cerebellar lesions.

PUPILLARY LIGHT REFLEX (A II → III REFLEX)

Each eye should be examined in room lighting for pupil size, shape, and symmetry. The size of the resting pupils reflects a tonic balance between the ambient lighting (parasympathetic input causing pupil constriction) and the anxiety or fear in the patient (sympathetic system). The resting equine pupil in room light is a horizontal oval that assumes a round shape when dilated (compare the pupils in **Figs. 1 and 2**). Pupil response to light should be assessed using *bright,* non-LED light. All observations should be repeated in a dark environment. Evidence of intraocular disease should be noted before interpreting the pupillary light reflex (PLR) as many ocular diseases such as uveitis, glaucoma, synechiae, and altered lens positions affect pupil size, shape, and response. Pupil sizes in the left and right eyes should be symmetrical unless there is significant color dilution in one eye ("blue eyes" are usually slightly more dilated). The PLR is a subcortical reflex that requires an intact retina, optic nerve (cranial nerve II), optic chiasm where the majority of nerve fibers cross to the contralateral side, to optic tracts in the diencephalon that course over the lateral geniculate nucleus in the thalamus, to the pretectal nucleus in the midbrain. Some fibers synapse on the ipsilateral parasympathetic (PS) lower motor neuron fibers but the majority cross to the opposite side to synapse on the contralateral PS oculomotor nucleus. The PS fibers then join their respective cranial nerve III (oculomotor) for a short distance while they exit the skull together. Once in the orbit, the PS fibers synapse in the ciliary ganglion and then travel to the eye along the optic nerve surface, eventually reaching the ciliary body and pupil constrictor muscles.[1(p169)]

To assess the PLR, dim the ambient lighting, ensure that both eyes dilate equally and symmetrically in the dimmed light and, using due caution in nervous patients, hold a bright focused light as described earlier approximately 2 cm from the cornea, directed slightly temporally in the eye toward the area centralis. Pupil constriction in both eyes is the expected result, with the stimulated eye constricting quicker and more completely than the opposite eye, noting that the equine and other ungulate pupils normally constrict more slowly than humans and carnivores. An observer on the opposite side can assess the response in the opposite eye or swinging light assessment can be performed (see later). If the light is maintained on the stimulated eye until full pupil constriction is obtained, a slight dilation or "pupil release" may then be noted. This is called hippus and is normal. The test is then repeated on the opposite side. In general, if vision and menace responses are normal and the direct PLR is normal in each eye, there is no reason to assess consensual responses.

A much simpler way to assess PLR integrity in the large animal patient, especially helpful when an observer is not able to assess the opposite pupil, is to perform a *swinging light test*. Stimulate one eye as described above, keeping the light close to the eye, directed temporally. Wait 5 to 10 seconds until both pupils have had sufficient time to constrict. Rapidly swing the light to the same position in the opposite eye. Repeat this several times, fairly quickly. Normally, the second eye should still be almost fully constricted from stimulation of the first eye and both should remain so as the light moves quickly from one eye to the other. If the pupil in the second eye dilates after the light swings to it, then there is an afferent pathway lesion in the second eye (retina, optic nerve, optic chiasm, etc.). If the second eye was already dilated when the light reached it, a parasympathetic denervation may be present in the second eye (parasympathetic fibers traveling with cranial nerve III) or an afferent pathway lesion is present in the first eye. If the stimulated eye fails to constrict, then an afferent pathway deficit or a parasympathetic lesion is present in the stimulated eye. The test should be repeated from the beginning on the second eye. Refer to **Table 1** for further details.

DAZZLE OR SQUINT REFLEX (A II → VII REFLEX)

The dazzle reflex is the blink or eyelid closure that may occur in one or both eyes when a very bright light is suddenly directed into either eye. A positive dazzle reflex indicates that the subcortical visual pathway and pathways to the facial nucleus and eyelid is intact.[1(p400)]

CORNEAL REFLEX (A V → VII REFLEX)

The corneal reflex is a subcortical V → VII reflex but there is no reason to assess the corneal reflex in most patients as the ophthalmic branch of V can be assessed in other, less uncomfortable, ways (palpebral reflex, nasal septum sensation). The afferent pathway is via the ophthalmic branch (V_1) of the trigeminal nerve (V). The reflex is elicited by very gently touching the cornea with a moistened cotton swab or a clean, moist fingertip. In addition to blinking in response to the touch (a normal V → VII reflex), the patient may retract the globe, indicating that the cranial nerve VI, the abducent or abducens nerve, is intact.

VISION TESTING

Vision can be assessed by observing the patient at work or by information obtained from the horse's handlers; these are unreliable at best but are often the reason for presentation to an ophthalmologist or neurologist. Vision assessment in a clinical setting is via observation of the patient moving on a loose lead line into the building, noting head carriage and ease while moving, etc. Obstacle course assessments can also be performed which should include alternately blindfolding each eye after nonblindfolded observation. Due caution should be taken in every setting to avoid injury to the patient and handler when blindfolds are placed, in part because vestibular and cerebellar diseases may worsen when the visual input to those systems is reduced.

AUTONOMIC INNERVATION AND THE EYE

The autonomic nervous system with its sympathetic and PS divisions is an entirely motor system known as the visceral efferent system. PS motor innervation to the eye effects pupil constriction as well as other functions and the PS pathway of innervation to the eye travels with cranial nerve III. Sympathetic motor innervation to the eye effects dilation of the pupil as well as other less obvious functions and the sympathetic pathway is quite complex. Loss of sympathetic innervation to the eye can occur secondary to a lesion anywhere along the sympathetic pathway from the head to the eye (brainstem → right and left side intermediate horn of spinal cord → ventral horn of the first few thoracic spinal cord segments → ventral roots and T1-T3 spinal nerves bilaterally → rami communicantes → cranial thoracic sympathetic trunks → through the cervicothoracic and middle cervical ganglia to the continuation of the sympathetic trunks up the neck). In the head, synapse occurs in the cranial cervical ganglion located caudomedial to the tympanic bullae adjacent to the dorsal guttural pouch mucosa and postganglionic fibers then travel with vessels and other nerves to their terminal locations in the eye (iris dilator and ciliary body muscles in the eye, circular smooth muscle fibers in the periorbital connective tissue and Mueller's muscle (orbitalis muscle) in the eyelid) as well as to smooth muscles in blood vessels and to the sweat glands in the skin of the head and cranial cervical area.[1(p173)] Postganglionic sympathetic fibers are *not* present in the middle ear cavity of horses (otitis media in the horse does not result in clinical evidence of sympathetic denervation).[1(p173)] In many animals, the most obvious signs of loss of sympathetic innervation to the eye (Horner or Horner's syndrome) are ptosis, enophthalmos, and miosis of the denervated side resulting in aniso-coria, which is most obvious in the dark (but which can be missed if pupil symmetry and size are not assessed in the dark). In the horse, Horner's is more easily diagnosed than in other species because of the excessive sweating that occurs secondary to the increased skin temperature that occurs when the sympathetically denervated blood vessels in the skin dilate. The eyelashes in the affected eye point ventrally due to loss of tone in the *arrectores ciliorum* muscles[2] (**Fig. 3**). Closer observation of the ipsilateral eye generally discloses only a mild ptosis and mild relative miosis when the patient is in the dark. Enophthalmos, nictitans prolapse, and conjunctival hyperemia seen in other species are also subtle in the equine patient. Nasal mucosal hyperemia and congestion may result in an increase in sinus nasal discharge and nasal congestion.

Because of the clinically obvious sweating in the equine patient, sympathetic pathway lesion localization is often significantly easier than in other species. If the patient presents with sweating of the entire face and head or localized facial sweating,

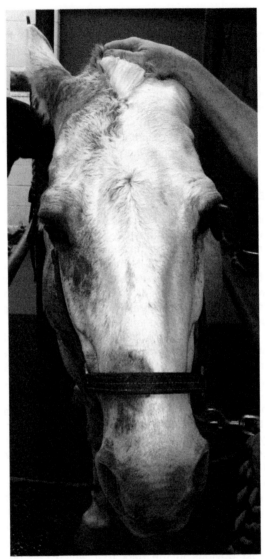

Fig. 3. A 23-year-old Missouri fox trotter gelding with right-sided Horner's syndrome. Note the hemifacial sweating and the markedly dropped eyelash angle in the affected right eye, findings typical of Horner's syndrome in an equine patient (see **Fig. 4**).

this suggests a postganglionic disruption of the sympathetic pathway such as might occur with guttural pouch disease, surgery, neoplasia, basisphenoid and other trauma, and so on. Sweating of the head and cranial 20% of the neck (up to the level of the second cervical vertebrae) suggests that the preganglionic sympathetic trunk has been disrupted near the guttural pouch or somewhere in the neck, possibly secondary to neck trauma, neck infections, severe choke and its sequelae, or as a result of an irritant injected perivascularly during jugular venipuncture. Sweating of the entire ipsilateral neck without other neurologic signs points to a lesion near the origin of the vertebral

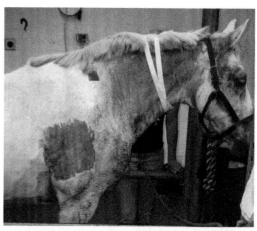

Fig. 4. Right side of the same patient shown in **Fig. 3**. Note sweating of the entire right side of the neck and cranial shoulder. Close observation of the clipped area caudal to the shoulder shows a sharply demarcated line of hyperemic skin consistent with the area of sweating. With the leg protracted cranially, a right-sided cranial thoracic melanoma was diagnosed on ultrasound-guided biopsy. A portion of the cervicothoracic ganglion, right vertebral nerve, and a few brachial plexus nerves were found at necropsy to be compressed by the mass.

nerve, in which case cranial thoracic imaging is strongly recommended (the vertebral nerve carries postganglionic sympathetic innervation from the cervicothoracic ganglia to the entire cervical region caudal to the second cervical vertebrae) (**Fig. 4**; see **Fig. 3**). Although described in other species to diagnose pre- versus postganglionic Horner's syndrome, pharmacologic testing of the eye to assess the denervation hypersensitivity associated with postganglionic lesions has little point in the equine patient because lesion location is usually more obvious than in other species. Administration of 0.5% phenylephrine to the affected eye, however, may help diagnostically in cases of orbital or retrobulbar Horner's where the only signs may be conjunctival hyperemia and/or altered pupil function with or without dropped eyelashes and may help to confirm a diagnosis of grass sickness in suspect cases (see later).[2–4]

THE VESTIBULAR SYSTEM AND THE EYE

The normal, centered position of the globes in each orbit depends on normal structure and function of both globes, adjacent connective tissues, extraocular muscles, the innervation to those muscles (cranial nerves III, IV, and VI), and the vestibular components of the vestibulocochlear nerve (VIII), all of which affect the control, position, and movement of the globe through pathways and mechanisms too detailed to discuss here. The routine examination a clinician must make to assess these nerves requires careful, general observation followed by a few simple head movements. First, with the horse's head in neutral position, check to see if any strabismus is present. Strabismus that is "down and out" (ventrolateral) is associated with cranial nerve III lesions while an "up and in" gaze (dorsomedial) is usually due to a cranial nerve IV lesion; a medial strabismus may be due to a cranial nerve VI lesion. Next, move the patient's head side-to-side while watching for the normal medial and lateral movements of the globe (saccades) that occur with head movement. If the globe being observed can move medially then the motor portion of III and the medial rectus muscle are normal. If the globe can move laterally, then the abducent nerve (VI) and lateral rectus muscle are functioning. If nystagmus is present in any head position, the vestibular portion of cranial nerve VIII is diseased. Peripheral VIII lesions are usually associated with rotatory or horizontal nystagmus (fast phase away from the side of the lesion) while central vestibular lesions can create nystagmus of any sort (rotatory, vertical, horizontal) with the fast phase being inconsistent. Blindfolding a horse with suspected neurologic disease should be done with caution as loss of visual input may cause dramatic worsening of vestibular signs and balance.

SUDDEN BLINDNESS IN THE HORSE: SELECTED CAUSES

Acute loss of vision in both eyes is usually recognized immediately as the patient is nervous, fearful, and unable to negotiate its normal environment. Unilateral blindness, especially of the horse's right eye, may be recognized only after the horse is noted spooking or bumping into objects on one side. In every case, a complete neuro-ophthalmologic examination is warranted, with close attention paid to pupillary light response, vestibular eye movements, and palpebral reflexes. The globe should be thoroughly examined with special attention paid to the fundic exam.

Acute, unilateral blindness can be seen after trauma to the eye or head, secondary to primary ocular diseases such as acute uveitis, corneal edema/hydrops, acute cataract, retinal detachments, and so on or with retrobulbar diseases such as optic neuritis, and space-occupying, compressive orbital lesions. Many of these conditions are chronic ones, but blindness can occur acutely. These conditions are not discussed here.

Examination of the acutely blind patient begins with a general inspection of head, neck and body for evidence of trauma or other abnormalities followed by a general inspection of both globes to ensure proceeding with an examination will not cause further damage to the eyes. In some cases, a known trauma has occurred and the subsequent exam can be focused accordingly. In all cases, the nostrils and ears should be checked for discharge, hemorrhage, and symmetry. Careful palpation of all skull bones for pain, symmetry, and swelling should be performed and sinuses should be percussed. Cranial nerves should be assessed as described above including the palpebral reflex, PLR, and vestibular eye movements. Menace response in several fields should be assessed. Each globe should be retropulsed to assess orbit swelling and nictitans movement. Intraocular pressure should be assessed in both eyes. Endoscopy of the upper airway should be performed including inspection of the ethmoid region and the guttural pouches. Depending on initial findings and laboratory evaluation, advanced imaging is often indicated.

Sudden Blindness After Head Trauma

Equine head trauma patients vary considerably at presentation but a common presentation is the equine patient that, due to tying, fear, or another reason, hyperextends its head during rearing and "flips over backwards." These patients, often blind immediately, will in most cases remain so forever. Other cases may develop visual deficits over hours to days following the trauma. In all cases, mild to severe vestibular and other neurologic signs may be present according to the extent and site of lesions present.

The pupils in the acutely blind post-trauma patients are variably dilated but may be fixed and unresponsive; menace responses and dazzle reflexes are variable to absent. In most cases the remainder of the ophthalmic examination is initially normal because the site of the injury to the optic nerve is several centimeters from the globe; between 1 and 2 months post-injury retrograde optic nerve degeneration has progressed sufficiently that optic nerve atrophy becomes evident on fundus exami-nation (mild to extreme pallor of the nerve head, reduced to absent retinal vessels, and segmental to extensive prominence of the lamina cribrosa of the optic nerve head).

Blindness in these cases may be due to shearing or severing of the optic nerves as the brain moves away from the fixed, intracanilicular optic nerves. In other cases, the nerves or optic chiasm are compressed by hemorrhage secondary to presphenoid or basispenoid fracture, by direct bony compression from fracture fragments, or by compression to the nerves from hemorrhage into the sphenopalatine sinuses. The basal skull fractures likely occur secondarily to excess rectus capitus muscle tension that occurs when the extreme head hyperextension during rearing creates undue traction on the synchondrosis between the basioccipital and basisphenoid resulting in a fracture.

Workup in these patients should include a complete neurologic examination, advanced imaging (computed tomography [CT] and/or magnetic resonance imaging [MRI]), and possibly cerebrospinal fluid analysis if the condition of the patient permits general anesthesia. Treatment is as for any central nervous system trauma. Prognosis for return of vision is generally hopeless. The few patients without fractures who retain some vision and pupillary function immediately after the injury may have visual acuity improvement over 2 to 4 weeks but, as stated earlier, return of vision is extremely unlikely in patients who become blind at the time of the injury.

Compressive Optic Neuropathy

Infections, inflammation, granulomas, or neoplasias in the thin-walled sphenoid and palatine sinuses (SPS) can result in blindness that may appear acute in onset or may be slowly progressive with a variable presentation. Advanced cases may present with visual deficits, bilaterally dilated unresponsive pupils, and optic nerve atrophy. Earlier in the disease course, the owner may complain of vague visual deficits and nervousness or other unusual behaviors; the PLR, optic nerve, and fundus examina-tion at that time may be completely normal. Visual deficits and pupillary light responses may wax and wane in some cases, especially in response to anti-inflammatory therapy[5] (Tom Divers, Ithaca, NY, personal communication). Cases with SPS mass or inflammatory lesions may manifest abnormalities of cranial nerves III, IV, V, and VI as these optic nerves are located immediately lateral to the SPS (the optic nerves located immediately dorsal to the sinus), but the optic nerves alone are affected more commonly.[6] Respiratory infections and chronic sinusitis are reported historically in some cases while other horses have no significant history.[6] A complete neuro-ophthalmologic examination is warranted in all cases. The ophthalmic exam, including PLR, vision testing, and optic nerve evaluation, may be normal, while other patients are blind with abnormal PLR. A complete hematologic examination is warranted. Advanced imaging modalities such as CT or MRI are required for diagnosis as the SPS is not accessible to endoscopic examination.[3] Sinoscopic biopsy can be performed in some cases, however.[7] As for acutely blind patients with a diagnosis of optic nerve compressive disease from any cause, patients with optic nerve compression due to SPS diseases benefit from immediate decompressive surgery but such procedures are unlikely to restore vision to animals blind for more than a few days. Prognosis and further treatment vary with the cause of the compressive disease. An adult warmblood presented with a 2-week history of visual impairment. The patient had no functional vision at the time of presentation but retained light perception, intermittent PLR, and dazzle reflexes. SPS sinus decom-pression surgery to expose the optic nerves and chiasm was performed and the patient remains stable and otherwise healthy 2 years later although optic nerve atrophy is present and markedly reduced vision persists (Normand Ducharme, Cornell University, Ithaca, NY, personal communication).

Ischemic or Blood Loss Optic Neuropathy

Bilateral blindness attributed to ischemia can occur after prolonged severe hypotension or hypovolemia in the horse. Prognosis is generally grave, although rare cases will regain vision. Acute ipsilateral blindness can occur in horses after inadvertent intracarotid injections, after arterial occlusion for treatment of guttural pouch mycosis, or due to thromboembolism associated with guttural pouch mycosis or other causes. Ophthalmic examination includes an afferent pupil deficit in the affected eye(s) ipsilateral to vessel ligation with a normal fundus exam or fundus examination may reveal optic nerve head pallor with or without retinal edema and hemorrhages in some cases. One case followed for several years by the author had blindness and no electrical activity detected in the retina via electroretinography after vessel occlusive procedures related to guttural pouch mycosis but regained functional vision in the eye between the fifth and sixth month postoperatively (electroretinogram also improved).

Optic Neuritis

The optic nerve collects the axons of the retinal ganglion cells after their course through the retinal nerve fiber layer and conducts them out of the eye toward the CNS at the optic nerve head. Immediately after leaving the eye, the optic nerve, like the rest of the central nervous system, is surrounded by three layers of meninges and contains cerebrospinal fluid. Thus, many diseases that affect the central nervous system can extend along the optic nerves and manifest in the eye including bacterial, viral, parasitic, or fungal meningitis and other diseases. The optic nerve in these cases may appear hazy and edematous and the normal lamina cribrosa detail that is always present in the horse may be absent. No cases of optic nerve head protrusion into the vitreous have been reported in the horse. The peripapillary retinal vessels may be swollen and hemorrhages may be present; retinal edema is usually present in the peripapillary retina. Affected patients may be completely or partially blind, and the menace response will vary accordingly, as will the PLR. Optic neuritis is also seen in some cases of equine recurrent uveitis, although the pathophysiology of the lesion is not clear. Complete neurologic exam is indicated coupled with electroretinography to confirm a functional retina, cerebrospinal fluid sampling, and CT/MRI. Treatment is directed at the cause if one can be found and otherwise steroids are used with caution. Prognosis varies according to the disease, duration, and response to treatment.

Toxic Neuropathy

This was the presumed cause of blindness reported 24 hours after pyrantel embonate administration to an anemic 10-month-old equine patient for treatment of *Strongylus vulgaris*. The eyes were normal ophthalmoscopically at the onset of blindness although the pupils were widely dilated and nonresponsive; palpebral reflexes were reported absent as well. When examined postmortem, 3.5 months later, the globes remained grossly normal, the retinae were normal, but myelin and axonal degeneration and atrophy of the visual pathway from the retrobulbar optic nerves through the optic tracts were present; the lateral geniculate region, optic radiations, and visual cortex remained normal. Inflammatory changes were not noted and the absent palpebral reflexes were not explained.[8]

Ivermectin toxicosis was the presumed cause of depression, ataxia, muscle fasiculations and bilateral mydriasis, reduced PLR, absent menace responses, and apparent blindness that occurred 18 hours after routine dosing of three adult quarter horses. Two of the three recovered with supportive care while the third was euthanized with high concentrations of ivermectin found in its brain.[9] Other cases have been reported secondary to overdosing. Ivermectin toxicity may be more likely in foals and it should not be used before 4 to 5 months of age in young equids.

Chorioretinitis

Chorioretinitis that is acute, bilateral, and severe may be due to many causes and may present with blindness. The ophthalmic examination may show incomplete to absent pupillary light reflexes. Fundus examination is usually diagnostic with indistinct peripapillary retinal folding or radiation of a soft white-to-yellow color with retinal vessels not apparent or slightly engorged. Intraretinal or subretinal inflammatory cells and exudates may be present along with retinal or choroidal edema or both. Differential diagnoses include equine recurrent uveitis, uveitis of any cause, septicemia, trauma, equine herpes virus 1 and 4, cryptococci, and viral encephalitis.

Focal-to-multifocal, inactive chorioretinal scars are the most common abnormality seen in the fundus of horses. Lesions are commonly clustered in the immediate peripapillary, nontapetal fundus, but may be seen peripherally as well. The classic inactive lesion has a circular or linear pigmented center (retinal pigment epithelial hypertrophy) with a white halo (sclera that is visible because of retinal pigment epithelium and choroidal depigmentation or atrophy). Clinical descriptions such as bullet holes, bird shot, and pigment bars have been applied to these lesions.

Retinal Detachments

Retinal detachments are actually retinal separations: the inner nine layers of the neurosensory retina separate from the outer retinal pigment epithelial layer of the retina. Any number of causes of disruption of the metabolic "pump" activity of the retinal pigment epithelium can result in a focal-to-complete retinal detachment. Retinal detachments with retinal tearing (rhegmatogenous retinal detachments) can occur from congenital abnormalities, from blunt trauma, or from penetrating injuries to the globe (including planned surgical procedures). The ophthalmoscopic appearance of "looking down the throat of a morning glory" is consistent with a bullous or nonrhegmatogenous retinal detachment, while a floating whitish-to-gray curtain, possibly obscuring the optic disc, can define a rhegmatous retinal detachment. If anterior segment disease precludes fundus examination, ultrasound is usually diagnostic. Patients with acute bilateral retinal detachment may present blind or severely visually impaired; unilateral or partial detachments are often incidental findings. Thorough medical assessment and immediate medical and possibly surgical therapy in selected cases directed at reattaching the retina(s) are warranted and are covered in standard ophthalmology and medical texts.

Exudative Optic Neuropathy

This has been reported as a cause of peracute blindness with bilaterally dilated unresponsive pupils in middle-aged to older horses of any breed (the author has seen only males affected). Fundus examination shows a variable, asymmetric amount and distribution of white myelin-like material on the optic nerve margins and in the vitreous. Hemorrhages (choroidal, retinal, intraretinal) of variable size may be present. No cases have regained vision. The condition is fortunately rare and is of unknown

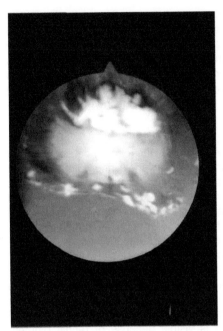 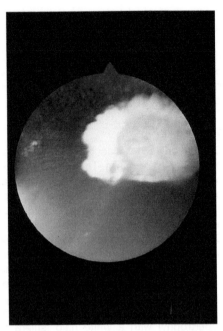

Fig. 5. The left and right eyes, respectively, of an adult stallion that was normal 2 hours earlier and found in paddock acutely blind. A complete medical workup and CT and CSF analysis were unremarkable. Large amounts of bright-white, myelin-like material was present at the margins of the optic discs OU, extending into the vitreous approximately 7 to 9 mm OS and 5 to 6 mm OD. Smaller clumps of a similar-appearing material were present suspended throughout the posterior vitreous of the right eye. Peripapillary retinal hemorrhages were present OS.

etiology, and reported cases have had no other significant disease findings. **Fig. 5** are ocular fundus images of a stallion seen at another institution and referred to Cornell for a second opinion after being found in the pasture acutely blind. There was no evidence of trauma and the horse was otherwise healthy on physical examination and on routine lab and endocrine evaluation. CT of the head and cranial neck was normal, as was cerebrospinal fluid analysis.

MISCELLANEOUS CAUSES OF CENTRAL BLINDNESS

Patients with focal to diffuse cerebral disease may have visual deficits or may appear totally blind. Many neonatal encephalopathic foals appear blind but are hard to assess because of their mentation and because young foals lack a menace response normally. Hepatoencephalopathy (HE) from any cause often results in reduced vision or blindness and many systemic diseases present with blindness as well as other clinical signs. If the patient can be examined safely, the patients do not menace normally but PLR and palpebral reflexes are normal. The eyes may have lid abrasions, corneal ulcers, or other lesions secondary to trauma associated with the often-severe neurologic signs. In addition to liver failure, HE may be seen with portosystemic shunts and a similar encephalopathy may accompany an acute colic episode secondary to hyperammonemia from overproduction of ammonia by gastrointestinal flora. The blindness is reversible if the primary problem or metabolic abnormalities can be corrected.

Central blindness can also occur in the postictal patient and may last for hours to days. Selected other causes of central blindness in the equine include equine protozoal encephalomyelitis (EPM), cerebral abscesses, leukoencephalomalacia, viral encephalitides, bacterial meningitis, cerebral trauma, and blindness after anesthesia and intracarotid injections (discussed later).

Postanesthetic Blindness

Postanesthetic blindness is a devastating condition of irreversible blindness, with or without other signs of cerebrocortical disease due to cerebral necrosis, that is believed to be secondary to decreased cerebral blood flow from one of many causes (hypovolemia, hypotension, vascular shunting) but due to unknown factors in many cases. The prognosis is extremely grave for return of vision. Five cases described by McKay and colleagues[10] developed signs between 5 hours to 7 days after the anesthetic episode; the cases had no apparent predisposing factors except that four of five were in dorsal recumbency, four of five had had colic, and all had elevated liver enzymes at the onset of blindness.[4]

Blindness has occurred in horses after myelogram procedures; all cases have regained vision within days (Tom Divers, Ithaca, NY, personal communication).

Blindness After Intracarotid Injections

Blindness after intracarotid injections may result in acute cerebral toxicity or infarction of the ipsilateral prosencephalon as medication travels from the common carotid to the internal carotid and then to the cerebral arteries. Contralateral blindness with normal PLR may occur. Decreased contralateral facial and corneal sensation after intracarotid injection has also been reported.[3,11]

MISCELLANEOUS CONDITIONS WITH NEURO-OPHTHALMIC CONCERNS
Facial Nerve Paralysis

Facial nerve paralysis can accompany central nervous system diseases such as EPM, viral encephalitides and otitis interna and may be seen with otitis media, temporohyoid osteopathy (THO), and peripheral damage to cranial nerve VII from any cause. Facial paralysis may present alone or in combination with other physical and neurological abnormalities. If only the palpebral branches of the facial nerve are involved, the patient will have reduced eyelid tone and ptosis and be completely unable to blink (although many patients appear to have partial blinks associated with drooping of the upper lid when the globe is retracted [abducent nerve and retractor bulbi muscles, in part]). If the entire peripheral nerve is affected, the presenting clinical signs may include ipsilateral ptosis, a deviation of the nose contralaterally and an ipsilateral ear droop; food boluses may be palpated in the ipsilateral cheek pouch. The ipsilateral eye should be examined carefully in every case of facial paralysis and should always include fluorescein dye and a careful examination at the time of presentation of the conjunctival and nictitans cul-de-sacs to remove any foreign material accumulation associated with reduced blinking. Schirmer tear tests (STTs) should be performed in every facial paralysis case (normal STT is >25 mm wetting/min); if Schirmer strips are not available, prior to instilling any liquid into the eye the clinician should inspect the interface between the lower eyelid and the cornea to assess the meniscus of tear film present there compared to the normal eye. Keratitis with or without ulceration, typically in the ventrotemporal third of the cornea, is often present at the initial exam and is secondary to reduced blink reflex, reduced tear film distribution, and decreased tear production in many cases. If ulceration is not present at the initial exam, it will develop rapidly in almost every case. Corneal ulcerations seen with facial paralysis are classic: horizontal oval-shaped ulcers just dorsal to the lower lid margin and slightly temporal on the cornea (the nasal and dorsal portions of the cornea are protected, respectively, by the increased nictitans movements seen in these patients to compensate for their lack of a normal blink and by ptosis of the upper lid). The ulcers often have a yellow-green discoloration and a dry, roughened, pitted surface. At the time of the initial exam, if the patient has facial paralysis and a reduced tear meniscus or a Schirmer tear test less than 10, a true ophthalmic emergency exists.

Every case of facial paralysis, with or without reduced tearing, should be treated as an emergency. Preventing corneal ulceration in these cases is much easier (and better for the patient) than treating an ulcer in a nonblinking, potentially dry eye because ulcers secondary to exposure keratitis rarely heal without moisture and without the protection of the eyelids. Such ulcers may worsen rapidly. Preventive measures should be instituted *at the time of the initial exam* and should include frequent lubrication with artificial tears and a temporary, lateral tarsorrhaphy. If a lateral tarsorrhaphy cannot be performed, then lubrication should be provided to the eye every 1 to 2 hours around the clock. Ulcer treatment should be implemented if indicated. Transpalpebral lavage (TPL) catheters, with or without a constant infusion pump, will facilitate lubrication in many cases until tarsorrhaphy can be performed. Once the lids are closed, ulcer treatment should be maintained as indicated either through the TPL or at the opened medial canthus. With the cornea now protected, and if no ulcer is present, artificial tear supplementation can be reduced to 4 to 6 times a day.

As the case workup progresses, if facial nerve function does not improve in the first 7 to 10 days, a more permanent solution is indicated to protect the eye over the long term, but this should *never* include enucleation as a therapeutic choice unless the globe is irreversibly damaged secondary to exposure keratitis. Temporary tarsorrhaphies are an ideal initial treatment, but sutures used to place them will fail over time and are otherwise problematic. In the author's experience, the vast majority of horses with facial nerve dysfunction will eventually regain normal eyelid function, although this can take as long as 18 months up to 6 years in one case. A reversible partial tarsorrhaphy is strongly recommended for lid closure until facial nerve function returns, at which time the adhesions that form between the lids as a result of the procedure can be incised and the lids restored to completely normal function and appearance.

Reversible tarsorrhaphies are of two types: simple intermarginal or split lid intermarginal. Simple intermarginal tarsorrhaphies, are performed after shaving or scarifying a paper-thin strip of tissue from apposing lid margins of the temporal two-thirds of the upper and lower eyelids and then suturing the scarified lid margins together with 6-0 absorbable simple interrupted sutures. In the author's hands simple intermarginal tarsorrhaphies generally failed after 1 to 2 months due to poor lid-to-lid adhesion formation. The author has used reversible split-lid tarsorrhaphies in 19 facial paralysis cases. In 14 cases where long-term follow-up was available, the patients have regained palpebral nerve function (2 months to 72 months, with the average return to function of 19 months). In all of these cases the thin layer of epidermis and conjunctiva that seals together the lids after the surgery heals is easily snipped open under sedation and topical anesthesia and adequate, extremely cosmetic eyelid function was restored in every case. The reversible, split-lid tarsorrhaphy is usually placed after the ulcer is stabilized, as ulcers can no longer be examined well after the lids are partially closed. Postoperative medications include topical antibiotic drugs or ointments applied three or four times daily at the medial canthal opening for 7 to 10 days. Lid swelling postoperatively is often considerable, but when the swelling subsides, if the eye was normal prior to the procedure, vision is usually excellent except in the far temporal visual field. Horses with reversible split-lid tarsorrhaphy have returned to full function if their health and neurologic status otherwise have permitted. Owners are asked to regularly assess the palpebral reflex; when it returns, the reversible split-lid tarsorrhaphy can be opened using sedation, topical anesthesia, and tenotomy scissors to incise the thin epidermal and conjunctival layer closing the lids. The procedure is explained to the owners as an "eyelid Caslick's," and once healed the procedures look very similar. Gaps may develop between suture sites but are of no concern and actually facilitate vision in the temporal fields. The technique for the reversible split-lid tarsorrhaphy has been described and illustrated previously.[12]

Keratoconjunctivitis Sicca

Keratoconjunctivitis sicca (KCS) is rarely reported in the equine patient and is usually of unknown etiology but has been seen secondary to facial nerve injury between the brain stem and petrous temporal bone where the parasympathetic fibers to the lacrimal glands travel with nerve VII. Cases have occurred secondary to petrous bone fractures with temporohyoid osteopathy but may also be seen associated with trauma more distally on the nerve or with chronic lacrimal gland inflammation. KCS combined with facial nerve paralysis can have devastating ocular consequences. All reported cases have been unilateral. Conventional medical therapy with or without a reversible tarsorrhaphy is recommended when parotid duct transplantation cannot be performed. An otherwise normal adult Connemara stallion that presented to Cornell with a 1-year history of bilateral chronic keratitis was diagnosed with bilateral, absolute KCS and secondary keratitis; his lacrimal glands could not be palpated and no other abnormalities were found after an extensive medical and endocrine evaluation. There was no history of previous lacrimal gland or orbital inflammation. CT of the head revealed no abnormalities but lacrimal glands were not seen. Nuclear scintigraphy confirmed that there was excellent flow from both parotid salivary glands, and bilateral parotid duct transplants were performed and were functioning well 1.5 years later (Keith Montgomery, DVM, and Sara McRae, personal communication).

Head Shaking

Head shaking is a frustrating and occasionally dangerous problem for owners, trainers, riders, and veterinarians. The patients throw their head at predictable or unpredictable times, sometimes to avoid certain activities and in other cases associated with light or transitions from bright light to shade and sometimes accompanied by snorting and nose flipping or rubbing. The problems sometimes worsen with exercise. There are numerous causes of head shaking and ophthalmic causes may include cystic corpora nigra, ciliary body or other uveal cysts, lens alterations, vitreal syneresis (resulting in vitreal "floaters"), retinal detachments, and optic nerve or other fundus masses (proliferative optic neuropathy or other). Other reported causes include otitis media/interna, sinonasal disease, dental disease, ear ticks or ear mites, sinorespiratory disease, and guttural pouch abnormalities. A very thorough workup usually includes detailed physical, neurologic, and ophthalmic examinations, skull radiographs, endoscopic examination of the upper airways and guttural pouches with attention dorsally in the area of the auditory fold as well as elsewhere, and careful dental examination followed by general anesthesia for a careful otoscopic examination followed by advanced imaging (CT/MRI). Treatment is

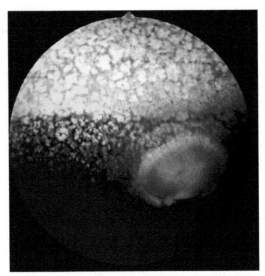

Fig. 6. An 11-year-old Connemara mare with signs of severe muscle weakness and with lattice-like, golden-to-dark brown lesions throughout the tapetal and nontapetal fundus of both eyes, was confirmed on postmortem examination to have equine motor neuron disease. Ceroid lipofuscin accumulation was found in the retinal pigment epithelial cells OU.

directed at the specific abnormality if one is found but in most cases nothing abnormal is found and patience on the part of the client is warranted as nonspecific interventions are tried sequentially. In these cases, fitted nasal masks, tinted goggles, tinted contact lenses, and opaque goggle over one eye (then later, the other) may be tried. Medical intervention with cyproheptadine, carbamazepine, melatonin, or other products can be attempted as can long-acting regional anesthesia of the infraorbital and ethmoidal nerve with neurectomy if response to the blocks is good. The prognosis is good if a cause is found but otherwise varies according to severity and response to treatment modalities.

SYSTEMIC DISEASES
Equine Dysautonomia (Grass Sickness)

This fatal disease, seen throughout northern Europe, the British Isles, and rarely in the United States, is a result of diffuse degeneration of the autonomic nervous system. The cause is unknown. Bilateral ptosis (markedly dropped eyelash angle but with normal lid tone) is one of the hallmarks of the disease, but other, much more dramatic, signs are variably present such as peracute, severe colic (impaction, gastric distension, displacements, other), tachycardia, multifocal areas of sweating, dysphagia, ptyalism, and so on. Chronic cases can develop severe weight loss accompanying other vague signs. A hallmark of many cases is patchy sweating, standing with all four feet close together, severely dry nasal mucosa, and bilateral ptosis. In suspect cases, dilute phenylephrine (0.5%) administered to one eye of an unsedated horse will result in return to normal of the eyelash angle in the treated eye compared to the untreated.[3] Specific diagnosis depends on histopathologic examination of autonomic ganglia in the gut or other affected tissues.

Equine Motor Neuron Disease

This disease is associated with vitamin E deficiency in horses and has a classic ophthalmoscopic appearance of golden-brown ceroid lipofuscin–laden retinal pigment epithelial cells distributed in a reticulated pattern. The lesions may be confined to the nontapetal fundus, concentrated along the tapetal-nontapetal border or distributed throughout the fundus (**Fig. 6**). All equine patients presenting with signs of vague lameness or weakness should have a fundus examination performed.

SUMMARY

A complete neuro-ophthalmologic assessment is relatively simple, requires minimal instrumentation and should be performed as part of every complete ophthalmic and neurologic examination. This article has summarized the tests that comprise and the species-specific details of the complete neuro-ophthalmologic of the equine patient. Selected causes of sudden blindness in the horse were summarized and some common neuro-ophthalmic conditions with significant ophthalmic consequences, such as facial nerve paralysis, were discussed. Split-lid tarsorrhaphies, which are indicated but rarely used in cases of facial nerve paralysis were strongly recommended for all facial paralysis cases and were described in detail.

REFERENCES

1. DeLahunta A, Glass E. Visual system. In: Veterinary Anatomy and Clinical Neurology. 3rd edition. St Louis: Saunders Elsevier; 2009.
2. Hahn CN. Horner's syndrome in horses. Equine Vet Educ 2003;15:86–90.
3. Mayhew IG. Neuro-ophthalmology: a review. Equine Vet J Suppl 2010;37:80–7.
4. Hahn CN. Miscellaneous disorders of the equine nervous system: Horner's syndrome and polyneuritis equi. Clin Tech Equine Pract 2006;5:43–6.
5. Barnett KC, Blunden AS, Dyson SJ, et al. Blindness, optic atrophy and sinusitis in the horse. Vet Ophthmal 2008;Suppl 1:20–6.
6. McCann JL, Dixon PM, Mayhew IG. Clinical anatomy of the equine spenopalatine sinus. Equine Vet J 2004;36:466–72.
7. Windley Z, Smith LJ, Bircham D, et al. The equine sphenopalatine sinus: assessment of normal anatomy by different diagnostic techniques and eight cases of primary sphenopalatine sinus disease. Proc 49th Br Equine Vet Assoc Congress 2010:233–4.
8. Kelly DF, Pinset PJN. Optic neuropathy in a horse. Acta Neuropathol 1979;48:145–8.
9. Swor TM, Whittenburg JL, Chaffin MK. Ivermectin toxicosis in three adult horses. JAVMA 2009;235:558–62.
10. McKay JS, Forest TW, Senior M, et al. Postanesthetic cerebral necrosis in 5 horses. Vet Rec 2002 (150) p. 70–4.
11. Mayhew, IG. Neuro-ophthalmology. In: Barnett KC, Crispin SM. Equine Ophthalmology. Second edition. London: Saunders; 2004. p. 251, 254.
12. Divers TJ, Ducharme NG, de Lahunta A, et al. Temporohyoid Osteoarthropathy. Clin Tech Equine Pract 2006;5:22–3.

Miscellaneous Neurologic or Neuromuscular Disorders in Horses

Monica Aleman, MVZ, PhD

KEYWORDS
- Horse • Junctionopathies • Motor neuron • Motor unit
- Nerve • Neuromuscular

Successful locomotion depends on the initiation and coordination of movement controlled by the nervous system over skeletal muscles. The peripheral nervous system can be classified into 2 major functional systems: afferent or sensory and efferent or motor systems.[1] The efferent system is comprised of somatic and visceral components.[1] This chapter will focus on the general somatic efferent system, specifically the neuromuscular (NM) region. The NM system is composed of motor units. The motor unit is defined as one lower motor neuron (or motoneuron), its axon and axonal terminal(s) or telodendron, NM junction, and all the skeletal muscle fibers (myofibers or myocytes) innervated by it (**Fig. 1**).[1,2] Briefly, there are 2 main types of motor neurons in the ventral horn of the spinal cord; A alpha (skeletomotor) and A gamma (fusimotor) motor neurons.[2] The alpha or extrafusal skeletomotor neurons have large cell bodies in the ventral horn of the spinal cord and fast myelinated conducting axons of large diameter located in the ventral root and spinal nerves.[2] Their axons terminate at the NM junction and only innervate extrafusal skeletal muscle fibers. The gamma or fusimotor neurons have smaller cell bodies and thinner, slower myelinated conducting axons that innervate intrafusal muscle fibers (muscle fibers contained within muscle spindle stretch receptors).[2] One-third and two-thirds of the motor outflow from the ventral horn are from gamma and alpha motor neurons, respectively.[3] There are also lower motor neurons within cranial nerve nuclei (III-VII, IX-XII) but will not be discussed here. Cranial nerve nuclei III, IV, and VI are discussed in the neuro-ophthalmic article.

A single lower motor neuron innervates muscle fibers contained within 1 muscle and not of different muscle groups.[2] The axon branches repeatedly to form a single NM junction for each muscle fiber innervated (see **Fig. 1**). Therefore, 1 muscle fiber is

The author has nothing to disclose.

Laboratories of Clinical Neurophysiology and Neuromuscular Disease, William R. Pritchard Veterinary Medical Teaching Hospital, School of Veterinary Medicine, Large Animal Clinic, One Shields Avenue, University of California, Davis, CA 95616, USA

E-mail address: mraleman@ucdavis.edu

Vet Clin Equine 27 (2011) 481–506
doi:10.1016/j.cveq.2011.08.001
0749-0739/11/$ – see front matter © 2011 Elsevier Inc. All rights reserved.

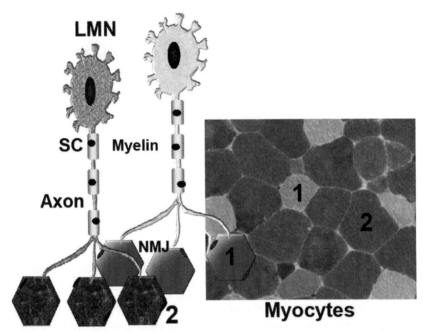

Fig. 1. Motor units (2), each composed of a single lower motor neuron (LMN), its axon, Schwann cells (SC produce myelin), neuromuscular junction (NMJ), and all the myofibers innervated by it. Note 2 LMNs independently innervating type 1 and type 2 myofibers. (*Inset*) Normal myofiber mosaic as shown on ATPase at preincubation pH 9.8.

innervated by 1 motor neuron. Large muscles (postural and locomotion muscles) on which fine movements are not required generally have a few hundreds to thousands muscle fibers per motor unit.[2] Muscles required for more dexterous movement such as those for ocular movement have fewer muscle fibers per motor unit (less than 20 in people).[2] A single discharge of a motor neuron will result in the contraction of all muscle fibers innervated by its axon.[4] All motor neurons innervating skeletal muscle are exclusively excitatory.[5] However, interneurons located within the spinal cord can have either excitatory or inhibitory effects on the motor neurons.[5] The neuron becomes depolarized or hyperpolarized if an excitatory or inhibitory stimulus predominates, respectively.[5]

The NM junction or motor end-plate is the region of synaptic contact of the following structures: (1) presynaptic membrane of the axonal terminal of the motor neuron, (2) synaptic space, and (3) postsynaptic membrane and junctional sarcoplasm of the muscle fiber.[5,6] Motor end-plates are located approximately halfway along the length of the muscle fiber.[7] The axonal terminal at the synaptic region has mitochondria and clusters of vesicles containing the neurotransmitter acetylcholine (ACh). Synaptic transmission from nerve to muscle involves electrical and chemical reactions.[7] The basic unit of neurotransmitter or quantum is the amount of ACh contained in a vesicle.[7] Upon depolarization of the presynaptic membrane and the influx of extracellular calcium, ACh is released via exocytosis into the synaptic space adjacent to the postsynaptic folds of the muscle fiber, where binding of ACh to specific nicotinic ACh receptors opens ions channels allowing Na^+ to move into the muscle fiber.[5,7] This generates an end-plate potential that can result into an action potential and contraction of the muscle fiber.[5] Acetylcholinesterase (AChase), present in the synaptic region, hydrolyzes ACh into acetate and choline. Choline is recycled into the presynaptic region and combined with acetyl-CoA for the formation of ACh.[6] For in-depth description of the anatomy and function of the NM system, the reader is referred to the first 6 references cited.

Neurotransmission can be modulated (inhibited or facilitated) by drugs and toxins. Its modulation can affect (1) peripheral nerve or presynaptic membrane, (2) synaptic space, and (3) postsynaptic membrane.[6] A few examples of drugs altering neurotransmission reported in people are shown in **Table 1**. Several of these drugs are also used in horses, some of which have been reported to alter NM function in the horse.[8-14] The clinician is advised to practice caution or avoid their use in horses with suspected NM disorder. Drugs affecting mainly the central or autonomic nervous systems are not included here.

NEUROMUSCULAR DISORDERS

This article will specifically discuss NM disorders involving skeletal muscle. Neuromuscular disorders are those affecting any component of the NM system and their supporting cells. Definition of a few terms will be provided for clarification. *Neuronopathy* is the abnormality of the neuron cell body, whereas *neuropathy* is the abnormality of the nerve. A nerve may be motor or sensory or both (this case both). Neuropathies can be characterized by degeneration of its axons (axonopathy), demyelination (eg, Schwannopathy), or both. *Junctionopathies* are disorders involving any of the presynaptic, synaptic, and postsynaptic regions of the motor end-plate.[6] Reported and suspected disorders affecting various areas of the NM system in horses are listed in **Box 1** and a few references are provided.[8,15-34] This article will describe a few disorders. Discussion of specific skeletal muscle disorders is beyond the scope of this text and the reader is referred elsewhere.[35-37]

Clinical Signs

The clinical signs will vary depending on the region of the NM system affected. Typically, lower motor neuron signs include generalized or localized muscle weakness (myasthenia), hyporeflexia to arreflexia, hypotonia to atonia, paresis to paralysis, and neurogenic muscle atrophy. Manifestations of muscle weakness include muscle fasciculations, low carriage of head and neck, standing with thoracic and pelvic limbs under the horse's abdomen, and toe drag. Disorders presenting with fasciculations include botulism, tick paralysis, equine motor neuron disease, equine protozoal myelitis, lead toxicity, electrolyte derangements, hyperkalemic periodic paralysis (HYPP), and West Nile virus. Muscle weakness can also be a cause of exercise intolerance. Reflexes including those involving cranial nerves may be decreased to absent. Depending on stage and severity of disease, not all signs of dysfunction may be observed. Gait deficits pertaining to specific nerves affected (eg, radial, femoral, peroneal, others) can be observed. Dysphagia, dysphonia, and dyspnea are also signs that should prompt the clinician to consider NM dysfunction (NMD) as a possible cause.

Signs caused by junctionopathies also vary depending on specific alteration: (1) location (presynaptic, synaptic, postsynaptic; (2) alterations in the production, release (increased vs reduced), binding, breakdown (increased by AChases, or reduced as in organophosphate intoxication [OP]), and uptake of ACh; and (3) specific ion channels affected at each location.[6] Examples of reduced release of ACh include botulism, tick paralysis, aminoglycoside administration, hypermagnesemia, and hypocalcemia (see **Box 1**).[6] Fluids containing magnesium can potentiate NM weakness in patients with botulism for example. Hypomagnesemia and black widow envenomation

Table 1
List of drugs associated with altered NM transmission

Drug Type	Presynaptic	Synaptic	Postsynaptic
Aminoglycosides			
Amikacin	+		+
Gentamicin	+		+
Kanamycin	+		+
Neomycin	+		+
Streptomycin	+		+
Anticholinesterases			
Organophosphates		+	
Edrophonium chloride		+	
Neostigmine bromide		+	
Pyridostigmine bromide		+	
Antiarrhythmics			
Class IA (Na$^+$ channel)			
Procainamide	+		+
Quinidine	+		+
Class IB (Na$^+$ channel)			
Lidocaine	+		+
Phenytoin	+		+
Class II (β-blockers)			
Propranolol	+		+
Class III (K$^+$ channel)			
Sotalol	+		+
Class IV (Ca^{2+} channel)			
Verapamil	+		+
Imidazole compounds			
Metronidazole	+		
Immunosuppresants			
Azathioprine	+		
Lincosamides			
Clindamycin	+		+ +
Lincomycin	+		+ +
Macrolides			
Erythromycin (enteric neurons)			
NM blocking agents			
Depolarizing			
Succinylcholine			+
Nondepolarizing			
Atracurium			+
Vecuronium			+
Pancuronium			+
Tetracyclines			
Oxytetracycline			+

(continued on next page)

Table 1 (continued)			
Drug Type	**Presynaptic**	**Synaptic**	**Postsynaptic**
Others			
Aminopyridines	+		
Anticonvulsants	+		+
D-Penicillamine			+
Lithium compounds	+		+
Polymyxin B	+		++
Procaine penicillin	+		+

+, Site of action; ++, predominant site of action.

result in increased release of ACh (see **Box 1**). Electrolyte derangements and OP toxicity (documented in humans) are examples of disorders for which more than one area of the NM junction may be affected (presynaptic, synaptic, and postsynaptic).[38] Lack of inhibitory input to lower motor neurons (eg, tetanus) results in rigid paresis or paralysis; whereas flaccid paresis to paralysis is seen with NM blockade and reduction or exhaustion of ACh (see **Box 1**).[6,39,40] Examples of presynaptic disorders characterized by flaccid paresis to paralysis are botulism and tick paralysis. Neuromuscular blockade can also occur at the postsynaptic membrane resulting in lower motor neuron signs as in the case of some snake envenomations.[1,34]

Myotonia is a common sign of myotonic disorders such as tick myotonia, myotonia dystrophica, and myotonia congenita.[41–45] These disorders are believed to affect muscle channels. Myotonia is characterized by sustained muscle contraction or delayed muscle relaxation after a muscle contraction. Myotonia can be focal, multifocal, or diffuse or spontaneous or induced by voluntary muscle contraction or muscle percussion. Other signs may include gait impairment, stiffness, muscle hypertrophy, and hypertonicity. Muscle atrophy and weakness can follow the previous signs in progressive myotonias such as myotonia dystrophica.[42]

A few disorders will be described in brief at the end to illustrate clinical signs. **Box 1** has a list of disorders classified under region affected of the NM system.

NEURODIAGNOSTIC APPROACH

Complete signalment and history are the essential first step in the investigation of any disorder. A history of a few or several horses affected in the same premises should raise suspicion of nutritional, toxic, or infectious causes. A thorough physical and neurologic examination must be performed for the evaluation of patients with suspected NMD. The reader is referred elsewhere for a comprehensive review on how to perform a neurologic examination in the horse.[46] Neuroanatomic localization is essential, and disorders that may present with clinical signs similar to those of NMD must be ruled out, particularly in the sick neonatal foal for which weakness, inability to rise, or apparent decreased muscle tone, among others, may be a common presentation for various disorders. Full blood work (complete blood count, chemistry panel, blood gases, and pH), and urinalysis should be part of a minimum data base collection. Although myopathies will not be discussed in this chapter, for purpose of clarification, muscle enzymes within reference values do not rule out a myopathic disorder (eg, HYPP). Neuromuscular disorders for which muscle enzymes may be

> **Box 1**
> **NM disorders reported or suspected in horses**
>
> Central
>
> Interneuron (Inhibitory: Renshaw cells)
>
>   Tetanus (*C tetani* toxins)
>
> Motor neuron cell body
>
>   Equine motor neuron disease
>
> Peripheral
>
> Neuropathy: mononeuropathy/multiple mononeuropathy/polyneuropathy
>
>   Anesthesia associated (compression, ischemia, hypoxia)
>
>   Drugs (cisplatin, colchicine, metronidazole, vincristine)[a]
>
>   Endocrinopathies/metabolic
>
>   Guttural pouch infection associated
>
>   Iatrogenic (drugs, alcohol blocks, neurolytics, postsurgical)
>
>   immune-mediated/inflammatory
>
>   Polyneuritis equi
>
>   Infection of adjacent tissues
>
>   Neoplasia (primary: peripheral nerve sheath tumor, secondary: lymphoma)
>
>   Neuroma (postsurgical)
>
>   Neuropathic pain
>
>   Recurrent laryngeal neuropathy
>
>   Toxic:
>
>   Arsenic
>
>   Lead
>
>   Ionophores (monensin, salinomycin, narasin)
>
>   Mercury
>
>   Organophosphates (delayed motor polyneuropathy)
>
>   Polyneuropathy of Scandinavian horses (presumed toxic)
>
>   "Stringhalt": *Hypochoeris radicata, Taraxacum officinal*
>
>   Temporohyoid osteoarthropathy associated
>
>   Trauma (eg, brachial plexus avulsion, "Sweeney")
>
>   "Stringhalt" (distal axonopathy)
>
>   Idiopathic, toxic, traumatic
>
> Presynaptic
>
>   *Reduced ACh release*
>
>   Botulism (*C botulinum* toxins A, B, C, D)
>
>   Drugs[b] (eg, aminoglycosides)
>
>   Hypermagnesemia
>
>   Hypocalcemia
>
>   Tick paralysis (females of *Ixodes holocyclus* [Australia], *Dermacentor* sp. [USA])

Increased ACh release

  Hypomagnesemia

  Envenomations (eg, black widow [*Latrodectus matans* α-latrotoxin])

Synaptic

  Drugs[b]

  Toxic (organophosphates: acute cholinergic, subacute intermediate syndrome, delayed motor polyneuropathy)

Postsynaptic

  Calcium derangements (hypercalcemia, hypocalcemia [eg, "tetany"])

  Drugs[b]

  Hyperkalemia

  Myasthenia gravis-like

  Hyperkalemic periodic paralysis

  Myotonic disorders: Tick myotonia (*Otobius megnini*), myotonia congenita/dystrophica

  Snake envenomation (rare: coral, rattlesnake)

Myopathy

  Noninflammatory

    Multiple subcategories

    Drugs (long-term steroids)

  Inflammatory

    immune-mediated

    Infectious

    Paraneoplastic

For more information about myopathic disorders and their classification, the reader is referred elsewhere.[35–37] Interneurons can have an excitatory or inhibitory effect on the lower motor neurons and therefore are included in this list.

[a] Drugs reported in people.

[b] See **Table 1** for a list of drugs.

elevated include ionophores, OP toxicity, equine motor neuron disease, and those associated with tick infestation.[8,15,45] Electrolyte analysis must also include ionized calcium (Ca^{2+}) and magnesium (Mg^{2+}) because these are physiologically active ions essential for NM homeostasis and function.[13,47] Alterations in pH may alter ionized calcium concentrations, since hydrogen ions (H^+) compete for binding sites on albumin and other proteins.[48] For example, alkalosis (increased pH [decreased H^+]) will result in less free calcium (Ca^{2+}). This change has been reported to be at a rate of 0.36 mmol/L per pH unit in people.[48] Cerebrospinal fluid (CSF) cytology is usually normal in NM disorders. Toxicologic screening of the diet, water, plants, soil, blood, stomach contents, feces, and body fluids including CSF may add useful or definitive information in suspected or exposed cases to toxicants. Consider imaging modalities such as radiographs, ultrasound, scintigraphy, computed tomography, and magnetic resonance imaging if indicated by a problem-oriented diagnostic approach. A full body necropsy and thorough evaluation of the nervous system by a trained neuropathologist

Table 2
Electrodiagnostic techniques for the investigation of neurogenic, neuromuscular (NM), and muscle disorders

Electrodiagnostics	Disorders
EMG	
Insertion	
Absent	Advanced or end-stage, nonmuscle tissue (fat, fibrous)
Prolonged	Denervated muscle, polymyositis
Spontaneous activity	
Fibrillation potentials (FP)	Neurogenic, NM, muscle
Positive sharp waves (PSW)	Neurogenic, NM, muscle
Complex repetitive discharges (CRD)	Neurogenic: motor neuron disease, muscle: HYPP, others
Myotonic discharges (MD)	Myotonic disorders: Myotonia congenita/dystrophica
NCV	
Motor	Various, lead toxicity, delayed OP toxicity
Sensory	Various, most toxic neuropathies
RNS	
Decremental CMAP	Myasthenia gravis (humans, small animals)
Decreased baseline CMAP	Botulism
Incremental CMAP (amp, AUC)	Botulism, hypermagnesemia (facilitation)
Incremental CMAP (amp only)	Nonpathologic (pseudofacilitation)
Mixed/multiple patterns	Organophosphate toxicity
SF-EMG	
Increased jitter	Junctionopathies

EMG = electromyography; NCV = nerve conduction velocity; RNS = repetitive nerve stimulation; SF-EMG = single fiber EMG; OP = organophosphates; CMAP = compound muscle action potential; Amp = amplitude; AUC = area under the curve.

are essential to avoid missing lesions. Neuroelectrodiagnostics are essential in the evaluation and diagnosis of NMD.

Neuroelectrodiagnosis

Neuroelectrodiagnostic medicine is considered an extension of the neurologic examination and refers to diagnosis based on the information obtained from neural conduction and electromyography (EMG).[4,6,49] Electroencephalography (EEG), brain auditory evoked response (BAER), electroretinography (ERG), EMG, single-fiber EMG (SF-EMG), nerve conduction velocity (NCV), and repetitive nerve stimulation (RNS) studies are examples of electrodiagnostic medicine. Applicable electrodiagnostic modalities for the investigation of NM disorders include EMG (including quantitative EMG), NCV, RNS, and SF-EMG (**Table 2**).[7]

Electromyography

Electromyography refers to the study of the electrical activity of the muscle. EMG has been particularly useful to detect disease processes affecting the motor unit (neural, junction, and muscular components).[50-52] The distribution of EMG abnormalities can assist in the localization of lesions to spinal cord segments, cell bodies of lower motor neurons, nerve plexus, and peripheral nerves.[50,51,53] Quantitative EMG can further assist in the determination of disorders as myopathic, neurogenic, or both.[52–55] While EMG does not provide a definitive diagnosis; its alterations can support or refute a diagnosis. However, EMG alterations are not pathognomonic of specific diseases.[50] For example, complex repetitive discharges are observed in horses with HYPP.[56] However, these discharges can be observed with other myopathic disorders. EMG can be performed safely in the standing horse with or without sedation depending on patient's cooperation, or under general anesthesia. In the author's experience, horses usually react more when testing distal limb muscles and sedation may be required. Depending on the muscles tested and duration of the study, the examiner may use short- or long-acting sedatives (xylazine hydrochloride [0.3–0.4 mg/kg IV] or detomidine hydrochloride [0.005–0.01 mg/kg IV], respectively). Advantages of obtaining EMGs in the standing horse include lack of alteration of muscle tone at rest (EMG at rest),[3] evaluation of the electrical activity of contracting muscle (EMG during activity) upon provoked movement by the examiner (eg, making the horse move its limbs or neck, bear more weight on one limb) or voluntary movement, and avoidance of possible risks of anesthesia. The study of EMG during controlled or sustained voluntary muscle contraction is routinely performed in the awake human patient but is not possible in veterinary medicine.

Insertional activity is that EMG activity related to mechanical stimulation of muscle fibers upon the insertion of the electrode into the muscle being tested. In normal individuals, this activity should stop within 1 to 2 seconds from insertion.[50] Spontaneous activity may be found at the end-plate or motor unit region.[50] Alterations of the EMG in NM disease can be observed during insertion or as pathologic spontaneous activity. Absent, decreased (low amplitude), increased (high amplitude), or prolonged (long duration) insertional activities indicate abnormality. Nonpathologic spontaneous activity can be seen if the needle is close to an end-plate(s) as miniature end-plate potentials (MEPPs) and end-plate spikes, or if a motor unit is detected as a motor unit action potential (MUAP).[2] The morphology (phases, peaks, turns), duration, and amplitude of each MUAP are important in the determination of abnormality and whether the disorder may be myopathic or neurogenic; for example, giant MUAPs are seen in neurogenic disease.[2,57]

Spontaneous activity reported in horses with NM disease includes fibrillation potentials, positive sharp waves, complex repetitive discharges, myotonic discharges, and neuromyotonic discharges.[8,51,53,56,58,59] In acute neuropathic disorders, EMG abnormalities may not be evident immediately.[50] It may take about 2 weeks to detect EMG alterations.[4]

Nerve conduction velocity

NCV studies assess the motor and sensory evoked responses to stimulation of nerves.[60] Motor nerve conduction requires stimulation of a nerve while recording from a muscle innervated by that nerve. Sensory nerve conduction requires stimulation of a mixed nerve while recording from a cutaneous nerve.[60] NCV studies aid in the localization of nerve, NM junction, and muscle disease. Furthermore, it aids in the distinction between axonal degeneration and demyelination.[60] NCV studies of the facial, radial, median, ulnar, lateral and medial palmar and plantar, sural, superficial, and deep peroneal nerves have been reported in horses and ponies.[27,61–69] These studies should be done under general anesthesia for safety reasons, patient cooperation, avoiding pain to the patient, and obtain interpretable recordings.

Most toxic neuropathies have symmetric clinical manifestations and are predominantly sensory.[70] Acute lead poisoning at high concentrations results mainly in a motor neuropathy in people.[70] Chronic lead exposure can cause both sensory and motor (predominant) neuropathies.[70] Neurologic manifestations of both motor and sensory alterations based on clinical signs (symmetric and asymmetric) have been observed in the horse.[31] Specifically, pharyngeal and laryngeal paralysis represents loss of motor function of pertinent nerves.

Repetitive nerve stimulation

This is the most commonly used diagnostic modality for NM junction disorders in human and small animal medicine.[7] A compound muscle action potential (CMAP) or M wave reflects the number of muscle fibers activated by a train of stimuli (repetitive stimulation) applied to a single nerve. The test is considered abnormal if fewer muscle fibers are activated during repetitive stimulation (usually 10 consecutive stimuli).[7] This is called a decremental response as seen in cases of myasthenia gravis.[71] The opposite, an incremental response of the M waves in its amplitude and area under the curve (more muscle fibers activated) is seen in cases of botulism.[72] Multiple patterns of abnormalities have been described in acute OP toxicity in people.[38]

Single-fiber EMG

This is a selective EMG for the study of junctionopathies by allowing the measurement of NM transmission of single end-plates.[6] The MUAPs from a single motor unit are recorded over a small area with a concentric EMG electrode. Variations in myofiber end-plate potential amplitude and firing threshold result in variations in latency of subsequent action potentials during nerve stimulation.[71] This phenomenon is termed NM jitter. Jitter is increased in diseases for which NM transmission is disturbed.[7,71] This technique has been scarcely used in veterinary medicine.[73–75]

Muscle and Nerve Biopsy

Muscle and nerve biopsy is an essential part in the investigation of NM disorders in various species by providing information on whether a disease process affects muscle, nerve, or both (**Fig. 2**). Histopathologic and histochemical alterations may not always be found in disorders affecting the NM junction; if present they are usually variable and nonspecific. The appropriate muscle specimen to collect will depend on the clinical condition of the patient. Any muscle can be collected in cases with suspected generalized or diffuse myopathies. Whereas in focal myopathies (eg, trauma, infection), the affected muscle must be collected to ensure a diagnostic specimen. This diagnostic modality can be performed in the standing horse by providing subcutaneous local anesthesia. Depending on patient cooperation and safety concerns, sedation may be required in some horses. The muscle biopsy should be obtained from an affected muscle but not so severely affected that it may preclude diagnostic interpretation (eg, excessive necrosis, fat or fibrous tissue). Ideally, the muscle should be one that has not been traumatized by injections or EMG studies. Muscle specimens approximately 1 cm long by 0.5 cm wide and 0.5 cm deep can be removed with minimal trauma and are usually cosmetically innocuous. Infiltration of local anesthetics and cauterization of the muscle sampled must be avoided. The best method for muscle collection is by an open surgical approach. However, other modalities such as punch biopsy for superficial muscles or Bergstrom biopsy needle for deep muscles such as the gluteus medius provide diagnostic specimens and avoid making larger incisions (**Fig. 3**). Complications secondary to the procedure are

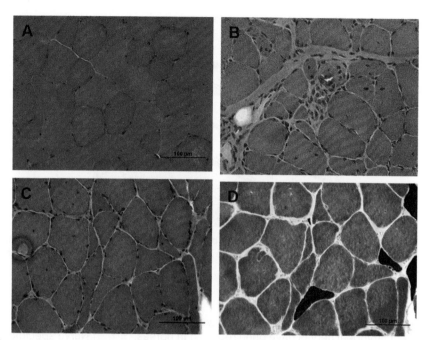

Fig. 2. (*A*) Normal gluteus medius. Note the polygonal shape of the myofibers and periph-erally located nuclei (hematoxylin-eosin, original magnification ×20). (*B*) Myopathy. Note centrally located nuclei, necrotic fibers infiltrated by macrophages (*center*) (hematoxylin-eosin, original magnification ×20). (*C*) Neurogenic muscle atrophy. Note anguloid-to-angu-lar myofiber shape (hematoxylin-eosin, original magnification ×20). (*D*) Neurogenic muscle atrophy and preponderance of type 1 myofibers. This is a sequential section of figure 2C on ATPase reaction at preincubation pH of 9.8 at original magnification ×20. Note anguloid-to-angular myofiber atrophy of both fiber types; type 1 = pink or light color and type 2 = brown or dark color.

rare but may include local swelling, hematoma, and infection. Tetanus toxoid vaccination must be current. The examiner is advised to contact the diagnostic laboratory prior to muscle collection to ensure that the specimens are properly collected, stored, and shipped. Whenever possible, collection of muscle samples for immunohistochemical fresh-frozen and formalin-fixed analysis is preferred. Determi-nation of fiber types, enzymatic reactions, protein assays, and immunologic staining can be performed in fresh-frozen specimens. Cells populations and morphology are best evaluated in formalin-fixed samples but could also be done in fresh-frozen samples. Muscle specimens must be collected in glutaraldehyde or modified Kar-novsky's for ultrastructural analysis depending on the laboratory's protocol. However, formalin-fixed specimens can also be prepared for electron microscopy evaluation.

Nerve biopsy samples are less commonly taken from horses compared to small animals due to relative unease of collection, safety concerns (almost always requiring general anesthesia), and possible complications.[76] For the same reasons, histologic, immunohistochemical, and stereologic studies of specific nerve specimens in horses have been performed immediately after euthanasia.[77,78] The selection of nerve to biopsy should be dictated by clinical basis, electrodiagnostic testing, and low morbidity. Fascicular rather than full-thickness nerve biopsy may reduce morbidity.[76,78] The surgical

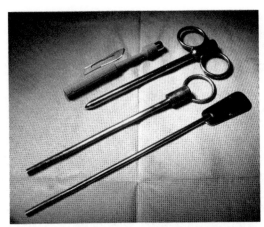

Fig. 3. Biopsy instruments for skeletal muscle collection. (*Top*) Scalpel blade and skin punch biopsy for superficial muscles. (*Bottom*) Three components of Bergstrom biopsy needle for deeper muscles.

approach for the collection of the spinal accessory, peroneal, palmar digital, and recurrent laryngeal nerves have been reported in horses.[20,78–82] Nerve specimens can be prepared for histologic, immunohistochemical, and ultrastructural analysis (**Fig. 4**). Semithin sections of nerve samples collected in glutaraldehyde can be plastic embedded and evaluated after toluidine blue staining for the quantification of large and small myelinated fibers, unmyelinated fibers, axonal diameter, axonal degeneration, myelin loss and splitting, and evidence of regeneration.[76] Single-teased fiber preparations can be processed from small strands of glutaraldehyde-fixed nerve to assess myelin internodes, demyelination, remyelination, and axonal degeneration in a single nerve fiber.[76,83] Evaluation of intramuscular nerve branches from muscle specimens provides useful information and aids in the diagnosis such as in cases of polyneuritis equi.[18] Ultrasonography can assist in the evaluation and collection of nerves.[18,84] However, this diagnostic modality has been underused in equine neurology.

NEUROMUSCULAR DYSFUNCTION IN CRITICAL ILLNESS

Acquired NMD in the critical care setting is a recognized problem in human medicine.[85] Since the establishment and advancement of state-of-the-art intensive and critical care units and training of specialized personnel in veterinary hospitals, it is important to note that NMD may also occur in our equine patients. Acquired disorders include critical illness myopathy (CIM), critical illness polyneuropathy (CIP), or a combination of both with a prevalence of 46% in critical patients.[85] These disorders are associated with sepsis, systemic inflammatory response syndrome, multiorgan dysfunction, or prolonged mechanical ventilation.[86] The clinical hallmark of NMD is weakness. Weakness is a common clinical sign in diseased neonatal foals, and recognition of acquired NMD may be challenging. As mentioned previously, ionized calcium and magnesium are essential for NM homeostasis. Disorders in the regulation of these ions resulting in hypocalcemia and/or hypomagnesemia have been reported in adult horses and neonatal foals with septicemia, endotoxemia, and gastrointestinal disease.[87–89]

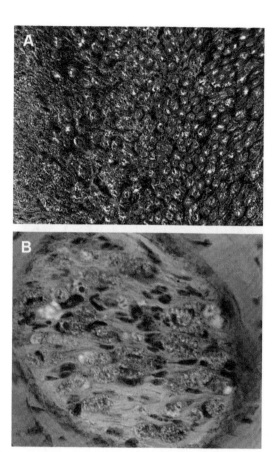

Fig. 4. (*A*) Fascicular nerve biopsy of normal superficial peroneal nerve. Note multiple axons (*dark structure* at the center of red staining) surrounded by myelin (*red staining*). (*B*) Abnormal intramuscular branch of the superficial peroneal nerve. Note the lack of axons and myelin staining. Both figures were stained with modified Gomori trichrome.

Identification and classification of NMD as CIM, CIP, or both require electrodiagnostic testing and histochemical and ultrastructural analyses of muscle and nerve.[86] A number of prospective studies have reported an increased risk of acquired NMD related to elevated plasma glucose levels, increased mortality associated with NMD in patients ventilated over 7 days, and prediction of mortality if NMD develops early in the course of critical illness.[85] Surviving patients may remain with long-term weakness and fatigue.

SPECIFIC MISCELLANEOUS OR NEUROMUSCULAR DISORDERS

The following disorders have been described in the literature; therefore, a brief description will be provided. References are listed for more information. Recent developments will be mentioned here.

Polyneuritis Equi

Polyneuritis equi (PNE), previously known as cauda equina neuritis, is an uncommon progressive neurologic disorder of undetermined cause that affects mature horses

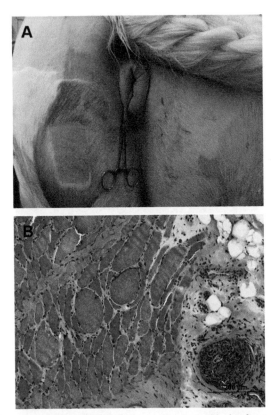

Fig. 5. Horse with polyneuritis equi. (*A*) Note anesthesia and lack of tone of anal sphincter. (*B*) Muscle biopsy of sacrocaudalis dorsalis lateralis on hematoxylin-eosin depicting severe inflammatory cell infiltration of intramuscular nerve branch (*bottom right above mark*) and neurogenic muscle atrophy. Cell infiltration is sparing muscle fibers.

and ponies (mean age 8 years).[90] The disease has not been reported in horses younger than 1 year. There is no breed or gender predilection. The disease is characterized by progressive, insidious granulomatous inflammation of the cauda equina and, less commonly, spinal and cranial nerves. PNE has been described in various breeds of horses and ponies with no apparent gender predisposition.[18,91–99] Most often horses present with insidious progressive deficits of the cauda equina such as decreased-to-absent anal and tail tone, loss of perineal reflex, and flaccid bladder and rectum resulting in urine and fecal retention and incontinence.[18,90,100] Cystitis and urine scalding can develop as a complication. Hyperesthesia of the tail and perineum, and sometimes the head, usually is the initial abnormality and progresses to hypoesthesia or anesthesia (**Fig. 5**A).[90,100,101] Severe cases can progress to involve other nerve roots in addition to those of the cauda equina and result in pelvic limb weakness, paresis, ataxia, and atrophy. In males, penile hypotonia, paresis, to paralysis may be observed.[18] Penile analgesia may occur since innervation to the skin of the penis is from the sacral plexus. Prepucial sensation is usually normal, though, since innervation of the prepuce comes from a more rostral area of the spinal cord (L3-L4). Signs pertaining to cranial nerve dysfunction (more common: V, VII, and VIII; less common: III, IX, X, and XII) may be seen.

CSF analysis may show variable and nonspecific alterations ranging from mild to moderate mixed mononuclear pleocytosis (predominantly lymphoid) with or without lymphoid reactivity, plasma cells (1 case), to primarily neutrophilic pleocytosis.[18,90] Protein concentration in CSF can be normal to increased. Collection of fluid from the lumbosacral site can sometimes be difficult due to "stricturing" of the dura at this site.

Extradural and, less commonly, intradural nerve roots of the cauda equina are thickened by granulomatous inflammation.[91] Lesions in the cauda equina tend to be more severe than those observed for cranial nerves.[90] Nerve fascicles appear demyelinated with subsequent axonal degeneration; thickened epineurium, endoneurium, and perineurium; fibrotic; and infiltrated by inflammatory cells including lymphocytes (T and B), plasma cells, lymphoblasts, macrophages, giant cells, and neutrophils.[18,90,94]

A diagnosis of PNE has been possible through a postmortem evaluation of the cauda equina and other nerves. Our laboratory reported a horse on which an antemortem diagnosis of PNE was reached through a muscle biopsy of the sacro-caudalis dorsalis lateralis.[18] This muscle showed a massive inflammatory cell infiltration of intramuscular nerve branches with sparing of myofibers (see **Fig. 5B**).[18] The infiltrates consisted of predominantly CD8$^+$ T cells and macrophages, followed by B-lymphocytes and plasma cells, and rare CD4$^+$ T cells.[18] These infiltrates were comparable to those found on postmortem evaluation that confirmed PNE.[18] The presence of CD8$^+$ T cells in excess to CD4$^+$ T cells supports an underlying immune-mediated process. Neurogenic muscle atrophy was found in this muscle.[18] Other muscles not innervated by nerves arising from the cauda equina were evaluated as controls and found to be normal. Circulating antibodies against P2-myelin protein have been found in some horses with PNE.[102] However, anti–P2-myelin antibodies have been reported with other diseases.[103] Ultrasound of extradural nerve roots and nerves may aid in the diagnosis.[18] Corticosteroids and azathioprine are potential treatments that might slow progression of the disease.

Botulism

Botulism is a potentially fatal flaccid paralytic disorder caused by the neurotoxins produced by *Clostridium botulinum*.[17] Eight antigenically distinct botulinum exotoxins have been reported to cause disease in various mammals, birds, and fish: A, B, C (C$_1$, C$_2$), D, E, F, and G.[17,104,105] Botulinum neurotoxins (BoNT) A, B, C, and D have been reported to cause disease in the horse.[105–109] *C botulinum* can be found in the soil and feces from herbivores.[17,110] Botulinum spores are resistant to heat but BoNT are heat-labile (destroyed at $>80°C$).[110] The disease has been documented in horses as sporadic cases and outbreaks.[17] The prevalence and type of BoNT causing disease vary depending on geographical location in the United States and throughout the world.[17,106–109,111,112] Type B is more common in North America, but types A and C have also been reported.[17] Type D is more common in South America and South Africa.[17] Types C and C/D have been reported to cause disease in Israel and Europe, respectively.[112,113]

Botulinum neurotoxins are 150-kDa single-chain polypeptides that consist of a heavy-chain (100 kDa) and light-chain (50 kDa) linked by a sulfide bond.[114] These neurotoxins are produced and released under anaerobic conditions, enter the systemic circulation, and migrate to the presynaptic membrane of motor neuron nerve endings, where BoNTs bind and internalize.[114] There is high affinity for the heavy chain at acceptor sites in cholinergic neurons.[115] Internalization of the BoNT occurs in a heavy chain receptor–mediated endocytosis.[115] Proteases in the terminal nerve ending cleave the heavy and light chains, releasing the light chain, which is the neurotoxic fragment of BoNT.[116] The light chain acts as a zinc-dependent endopeptidase that

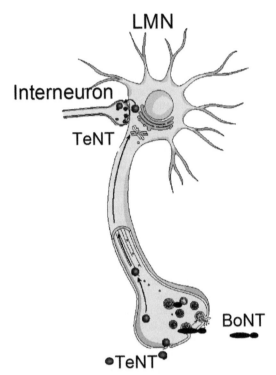

Fig. 6. Clostridial neurotoxins site of action. BoNT = botulinum neurotoxin; LMN = lower motor neuron; TeNT = tetanus neurotoxin.

selectively cleaves specific proteins involved in vesicle fusion.[116] Synaptosomal vesicle fusion requires the interactions of more than a half a dozen different proteins. Most strains of *C botulinum* can produce only 1 type of BoNT.[115] However, a specific BoNT can target 1 or more proteins.[39] Serotypes A, C, and E cleave SNAP-25 (synaptosomal-associated membrane protein 25), and BoNT B, D, F, and G cleave VAMP (vesicular-associated membrane protein or synaptobrevin).[104,115] Additionally, type C cleaves the membrane protein syntaxin.[115] The disruption of membrane fusion prevents the release of ACh into the synaptic cleft resulting in the interruption of NM transmission, which leads to functional denervation of the muscle. For sites of action of clostridial neurotoxins (tetanus neurotoxins [TeNT affects mainly Renshaw cells] and BoNT), see **Fig. 6.**

Clinical forms and signs
Clinically relevant routes of intoxication in horses include toxicoinfectious, food-borne, and, less commonly, wound botulism.[17,108] Toxicoinfectious botulism is the most common form of disease in foals younger than 6 months of age with the majority occurring between the ages of 2 and 6 weeks old and occurs when spores are ingested and then germinate in the intestinal tract.[40,72,108] In adult horses, the most common form is the food-borne botulism.[17,107,111] Equine grass sickness, a frequently fatal neurodegenerative dysautonomia in horses, is considered by some authors to be a toxicoinfectious form of botulism involving *C botulinum* type C (BoNT C_1 and binary C_2 produced locally within the gastrointestinal tract).[117]

Myasthenia, muscle fasciculations, low carriage of the head and neck (particularly common with BoNT type C), decreased suckle and drooling milk when suckling in foals, slow eating, dysphagia, dysphonia, decreased eyelid, tongue, tail and anal tone, mydriasis, decreased pupillary light reflexes (not always observed), exercise intolerance, constipation, and ileus are common signs in patients with botulism. However, onset and type of clinical signs, rate of progression, and prognosis vary from horse to horse, dose, and type of BoNT causing disease.[17,105,111,118] Lower doses (10^3 mouse lethal dose [MLD]) result in gradual onset and progression of signs over 5 to 10 days, and horses may develop transient signs.[17] Dysphagia may be an early sign in affected horses.[17] Transient dysphagia has been reported to be the only sign in mildly affected horses.[17] Larger doses (10^8 MLD) result in peracute, rapidly progressive disease that can result in recumbency within 8 to 12 hours of the first observed signs.[17] According to Whitlock, BoNT type C usually causes respiratory effort characterized by pronounced and prolonged abdominal lift rarely observed with other forms of BoNT.[17] In people, disease caused by BoNT type A is associated with more severe disease, longer recovery period, and higher mortality.[6,40] Similarly, botulism caused by BoNT type A in horses appears to be more severe and has a high mortality.[109] Disease with any BoNT can progress to recumbency, inability to stand, and death from respiratory failure. Complications associated with recumbency include pressure necrosis of the skin and muscles, difficult defecation and urination, inability to ventilate properly, and aspiration pneumonia. Pronounced muscle atrophy has been reported in a few surviving horses with botulism type C.[111]

Diagnosis

The diagnosis of botulism in most cases is clinical and by exclusion of other diseases with similar signs. The identification of C botulinum spores (gastrointestinal content, feces, wounds) or BoNTs (gastrointestinal content, feces, contaminated feed, serum) has a low yield.[40] However, spores of C botulinum type B are found in feces of 34% adult horses with disease.[17] Toxins and spores can be found in 20% and 70% of diseased foals, respectively.[17,108] Since the organism can be a normal inhabitant of the gastrointestinal tract, isolation of the pathogen in feces may be incidental. However, spores are rarely detected in feces from normal horses. Detection of neutralizing antibodies (anti-BoNT) through enzyme-linked immunosorbent assay may support botulism in unvaccinated horses.[112] The mouse inoculation test is the most reliable diagnostic technique in which protected and unprotected mice to specific botulinum antitoxin are injected with the patient's samples (eg, serum, gastrointestinal content, feces).[40] This test also determines the specific type of BoNT. More recently, novel multiplex polymerase chain reaction techniques have been developed for the identification of specific BoNT genes in tissues, food, and feces.[119,120] A singleplex qPCR for type B BoNT gene is available at the University of Pennsylvania (Botulism Laboratory, New Bolton Center, Kennett Square, PA, USA).

Although EMG is helpful in the investigation of NM disorders, it is usually normal in people with botulism. Further, the EMG can be abnormal in neurologic and muscle disease. Electrodiagnostics specific for NM junction disorders include RNS and SF-EMG.[6] We recently developed at our hospital a technique that proved to be useful and supportive of botulism in foals.[72] The technique is minimally invasive, requiring sedation of the patient, subcutaneous electrodes, and EMG machine that can perform RNS. Significant differences in CMAPs, amplitude, and area under the curve at baseline and in response to RNS at high rates of stimulation (50 Hz) were identified when comparing affected and healthy foals.[72]

Treatment and vaccination

For details of treatment, see article on toxic causes of neurologic disorders. In endemic areas, vaccination is indicated. Toxoids for *C botulinum* types B (BotVax B; Neogen Co, Lexington, KY, USA) and C/D (Botulism Vaccine; Onderstepoort Biological Products Ltd, Onderstepoort, Republic of South Africa) are commercially available. These vaccines are formalin-inactivated toxoids. Guidelines for vaccination are available at the American Association of Equine Practitioners (www.aaep.org). Toxoids for *C botulinum* types C and D have been used in the research setting but not licensed for commercial use in North America. More recently, monovalent and bivalent vaccines with recombinant heavy chain domain of BoNT types C and C/D (HcBoNT/C and HcBoNT/C and D) have been developed and used experimentally in horses.[121,122] Vaccination with HcBoNT induced anti-BoNT/C and D IgG similar or superior to those of horses vaccinated with available toxoid.[121] Local reactions at the site of injection were minimal.

Tick-Associated Neuromuscular Dysfunction

Tick paralysis and tick myotonia are different disorders and not to be confused with each other. They are caused by the neurotoxins produced by different ticks (paralysis in Australia hard ticks: *Ixodes holocyclus*, North America soft ticks: *Dermacentor* sp.; myotonia: *Otobius megnini*) that alter NM transmission at different sites (see **Box 1**).[33,45] Clinical manifestations of both disorders also differ (rapidly progressive flaccid paralysis vs myotonia). Tick paralysis can be clinically undistinguishable from botulism.[33] Dysphagia, decreased jaw tone, and laryngeal paralysis can be seen with tick paralysis. The ixodid ticks generally produce rapid and profound paralysis that can result in death due to respiratory failure within hours to a few days from infestation.[33] Muscle enzyme elevations can be seen with both infestations (tick myotonia CK 4,000–170,000 IU/L).[45] Hypertonicity, myotonia, and colic- and seizure-like signs are observed and can be induced by percussion in horses with tick myotonia.[45] Improvement of clinical signs for both disorders may take a few days after tick treatment or removal if not fatal as in the case of progressive paralysis.[1,45]

Hypocalcemia

Hypocalcemia in the horse can manifest as muscle fasciculations, colic and abdominal distention due to ileus, colic-like signs due to apparent muscle pain, sweating, salivation, synchronous diaphragmatic flutter, "tetany," high-stepping gait, trismus, tremors, seizure-like activity, seizures, staggering, ataxia, and recumbency. Signs in horses with moderate to severe hypocalcemia can be indistinguishable from those of tetanus (generalized muscle rigidity, stiff stance).[123] Laminitis must be ruled out since horses may present with lameness and stiff, short strides, and apparent pain that can resemble laminitis. Measuring plasma ionized calcium is essential to confirm the diagnosis. Total serum calcium does not reflect ionized hypocalcemia and severity. However, moderately to profoundly low total calcium with normal total protein and albumin supports hypocalcemia as the cause of signs. Electrolyte derangements and interactions with other ions can affect the function of the NM junction at different levels resulting in different clinical manifestations. History of recent ongoing severe rhabdomyolysis, late pregnancy, lactating mares, endurance rides, excessive sweating, bicarbonate treatment, and bisphosphonates administration should be investigated in horses with hypocalcemia. Rarely, persistent hypocalcemia may occur in growing foals. Other important causes of hypocalcemia include blister beetle toxicosis, acute renal failure, oxalate toxicity, and administration of tetracyclines, magnesium, and enemas with high content of phosphorus. Critically ill patients (adults and neonatal foals) such as those with septicemia and endotoxemia are more likely to develop calcium regulation disorders.[87–89] The opposite, hypercalcemia, can induce hypomagnesemia.[124] Hypomagnesemia is also observed in horses with critical illness and gastrointestinal disease.[87,125] Treatment of hypocalcemic tetany is slow administration of calcium borogluconate and correction of predisposing causes.

Organophosphate Toxicity

Three clinical forms of OP toxicity have been reported in people and suspected in horses.[8,38,126] These forms include acute cholinergic syndrome, subacute intermediate syndrome, and delayed OP-induced motor polyneuropathy.[38,126] Intoxicated individuals may develop 1, 2, or all 3 forms of toxicity.[38] Cholinergic dysfunction results in muscarinic, nicotinic, and central effects due to excessive accumulation of ACh at all levels of the nervous system.[38] Classically, OP intoxication presents with acute signs of muscarinic dysfunction such as salivation, lacrimation, increased urination, and diarrhea.[127] Nicotinic signs consist of transient rigidity, tremors, and weakness. Central signs include tremors and seizure-like activity. Intermediate syndrome develops within 1 to 4 days after the acute cholinergic crisis and is characterized by weakness, particularly of neck and postural muscles and muscles innervated by cranial nerves.[38,126] Respiratory failure resulting from weakness of the larynx and respiratory muscles is an important cause of death in intoxicated people.[38,126] Dysphagia due to pharyngeal weakness is also common. In this form, persistent inhibition of cholinesterases by OP results in presynaptic and postsynaptic impairment during NM transmission and calcium entry into myocytes causing myonecrosis.[126,128] Signs of motor polyneuropathy develop 1 to 3 weeks after OP exposure and consist of flaccid paresis and weakness of distal muscles.[38] Recovery from this form is usually poor in people.[38]

We reported 4 American Miniature horses with OP toxicity that recently received a complete-feed pelleted diet containing tetrachlorvinphos as a method of feed-through fly control.[8] These horses had been supplemented with vitamin E and selenium for the previous 8 months prior to the diet change. Signs developed within a few days from the diet change (diet containing OP). The signs consisted of diffuse muscle weakness, dysphagia, nostril flare, muscle fasciculations, low carriage of head, rhabdomyolysis, apparent muscle pain (myalgia; especially of the masseter muscles), reluctance to walk, lying down frequently, and decreased gastrointestinal sounds.[8] Whole blood cholinesterase activity in these horses was low (0.8–1.2 μmol/L/g/min [normal >1.7 μmol/L/g/min]). Elevations of muscle enzyme activities due to myonecrosis were also found (CK 385–176,418 IU/L, AST within reference to 34,848 IU/L). EMG in these horses was abnormal and consisted of fibrillation potentials and positive sharp waves. Horses received intensive supportive therapy and plasma as a source of cholinesterases. The only survivor was not presented at our institution since the signs were not severe. The rest of the herd did not receive the complete-feed diet and was clinically healthy. On histopathologic evaluation, all 3 horses had severe necrotizing myopathy of multiple muscles including respiratory muscles and, in 1, cardiac muscle. Ionophore intoxication was ruled out as the cause of such myopathy.

Treatment should be directed to (1) prevent further absorption of OP if recent exposure with gastric lavage and activated charcoal; (2) counteract muscarinic signs with atropine sulfate (caution as it can cause ileus), and nicotinic signs with pralidoxime hydrochloride to reverse binding of cholinesterase inhibitors with cholinesterases (use within 24–48 hours postexposure); and (3) provide supportive care. Plasma is a source of cholinesterases (measured at our institution from commercial plasma); however, its efficacy as an adjunctive treatment for OP toxicity is to be proved.[8]

Shivers

"Shivers" is a lay term given to the clinical manifestation of flexion and trembling of pelvic limb(s), trembling of musculature of pelvic limb(s), and trembling of the tail while held erect. Occasionally, other muscles may be noted to tremble, including facial muscles. Thoracic limbs may be involved but this occurs rarely. Shivering has been reported more commonly in draft and Warmblood breeds.[129,130] However, it has been observed in other breeds but less commonly. There is no gender predisposition and onset of signs can occur at any age older than 1 year. Signs may be noted or exacerbated when the horse moves, especially walking backward; coming out of the trailer; going into or outside stocks or confined areas; attempting to lift a foot by the farrier; while shoeing, changing, or walking on different surfaces; wearing a harness; and with excitement. With progression of disease, horses can develop muscle atrophy and weakness of pelvic limbs and another affected areas. Other common disorder in drafts and Warmblood horses is polysaccharide storage myopathy (PSSM).[129,130] Shivers and PSSM can occur concomitantly but no relation exists between the 2 disorders as proved by Firshman colleagues in a group of 103 Belgian draft horses.[130] In that study, the prevalence for shivers, PSSM, and both were 18%, 36%, and 6%, respectively.[130]

The etiology of this poorly understood disorder is unknown and the anatomic location remains undetermined despite full postmortem examination, electrodiagnostic testing, and evaluation of multiple muscle and nerve biopsies of affected limbs. It is possible that lesions have been missed (histopathologic evaluation not performed by neuropathologists) or the problem may be exclusively functional and not anatomic. Currently, there is no effective treatment for this progressive disorder (a few horses may remain static); therefore, the prognosis is unfavorable to poor. Since there is a breed predisposition, breeding out from affected horses has been considered. Medications, controlled exercise and rest regimens, and dietary modifications with high fat content have been attempted with variable results.

SUMMARY

NMD is an important cause of morbidity in horses. Signs of dysfunction could be variable depending on the specific area affected. NM disease can go unrecognized if a thorough evaluation is not performed in diseased horses. Electrodiagnostic testing is an area that has the potential to document and improve our understanding of NM disease yet is uncommonly performed. Keeping an open and observant mind will enhance our ability to search and find answers.

REFERENCES

1. DeLahunta A, Glass EN. Veterinary neuroanatomy and clinical neurology. 3rd edition. Philadelphia: Saunders Elsevier; 2008.
2. Dumitru D, Zwarts MJ. Needle electromyography In: Dumitru D, Amato AA, Zwarts MJ, editors. Electrodiagnostics in diseases of nerve and muscle: principles and practice. Philadelphia: Hanley & Belfus; 2002. p. 257–91.
3. King AS. Somatic motor systems: general principles. In: King AS, editor. Physiological and clinical anatomy of the domestic mammals. Malaysia: Blackwell Science, 2008. p. 131–40.
4. Kimura J. Electrodiagnostics in diseases of nerve and muscle: principles and practice. 3rd edition. New York: Springer; 2001.

5. King AS. Central nervous system. In: King AS, editor. Physiological and Clinical Anatomy of the Domestic Mammals. Malaysia: Blackwell Science; 2008.

6. Dumitru D, Amato AA. Neuromuscular junction disorders. In: Dumitru D, Amato AA, Zwarts MJ, editors. Electrodiagnostic medicine. 2nd edition. Philadelphia: Hanley & Belfus; 2002. p. 1127–228.

7. Sanders DB. Electrophysiologic study of disorders of neuromuscular transmission. In: Aminoff MJ, editor. Electrodiagnosis in clinical neurology. 4th edition. Philadelphia: Churchill Livingstone; 1999. p. 303–21.

8. Myers CJ, Aleman M, Heidman P, et al. Myopathy in American miniature horses. Equine Vet J 2006;38:272–6.

9. Hildebrand SV, Hill T. Interaction of gentamycin and atracurium in anaesthetised horses. Equine Vet J 1994;26:209–11.

10. Jones RS, Prentice DE. A technique for the investigation of the action of drugs on the neuromuscular junction in the intact horse. Br Vet J 1976;132:226–30.

11. Hague BA, Martinez EA, Hartsfield SM. Effects of high-dose gentamicin sulfate on neuromuscular blockade in halothane-anesthetized horses. Am J Vet Res 1997;58: 1324–6.

12. Nieto JE, Rakestraw PC, Snyder JR, et al. In vitro effects of eyrthromycin, lidocaine, metoclopramide on smooth muscle from the pyloric antrum, proximal portion of the duodenum, and middle portion of the jejunum of horses. Am J Vet Res 2000;61: 413–9.

13. Bowen JM, McMullan WC. Influence of induced hypermagnesemia and hypocalcemia on neuromuscular blocking property of oxytetracycline in the horse. Am J Vet Res 1975;36:1025–8.

14. Hildebrand SV. Neuromuscular blocking agents in equine anesthesia. Vet Clin North Am Equine Pract 1990;6:587–606.

15. Aleman M, Magdesian KG, Peterson TS, et al. Salinomycin toxicosis in horses. J Am Vet Med Assoc 2007;230:1822–6.

16. Hahn CN, Matiasek K, Dixon PM, et al. Histological and ultrastructural evidence that recurrent laryngeal neuropathy is a bilateral mononeuropathy limited to recurrent laryngeal nerves. Equine Vet J 2008;40:666–72.

17. Whitlock RH. Botulism (shaker foals; forage poisoning). In: Smith BP, editor. Large animal internal medicine. 4th edition. St Louis (MO): Mosby Elsevier; 2009. p. 1096–101.

18. Aleman M, Katzman SA, Vaughan B, et al. Antemortem diagnosis of polyneuritis equi. J Vet Intern Med 2009;23:665–8.

19. Franci P, Leece EA, Brearley JC. Post anaesthetic myopathy/neuropathy in horses undergoing magnetic resonance imaging compared to horses undergoing surgery. Equine Vet J 2006;38:497–501.

20. Armengou L, Anor S, Climent F, et al. Antemortem diagnosis of a distal axonopathy causing severe stringhalt in a horse. J Vet Intern Med 2010;24:220–3.

21. Bell C. Pharyngeal neuromuscular dysfunction associated with bilateral guttural pouch tympany in a foal. Can Vet J 2007;48:192–4.

22. Sturgeon BPR, Milne EM, Smith KC. Benign peripheral nerve sheath tumor of the perianal region in a young pony. J Vet Diagn Invest 2008;20:93–6.

23. Hanche-Olsen S, Teige J, Skaar I, et al. Polyneuropathy associated with forage sources in Norwegian horses. J Vet Intern Med 2008;22:178–84.

24. Hahn CN, Matiasek K, Syrja P, et al. Polyneuropathy of Finnish horses characterised by inflammatory demyelination and intracisternal Schwann cell inclusions. Equine Vet J 2008;40:231–6.

25. Toth F, Schumacher J, Schramme M, et al. Compressive damage to the deep branch of the lateral plantar nerve associated with lameness caused by proximal suspensory desmitis. Vet Surg 2008;37:328–35.

26. Schoniger S, Summers BA. Localized, plexiform, diffuse, and other variants of neurofibroma in 12 dogs, 2 horses, and a chicken. Vet Pathol 2009;46:904–15.

27. Huntington PJ, Jeffcott LB, Friend SC, et al. Australian Stringhalt–epidemiological, clinical and neurological investigations. Equine Vet J 1989;21:266–73.

28. Galey FD, Hullinger PJ, McCaskill J. Outbreaks of stringhalt in northern California. Vet Hum Toxicol 1991;33:176–7.

29. Crabill MR, Honnas CM, Taylor DS, et al. Stringhalt secondary to trauma to the dorsoproximal region of the metatarsus in horses: 10 cases. J Am Vet Med Assoc 1994;205:867–9.

30. Domange C, Casteignau A, Collington G, et al. Longitudinal study of Australian stringhalt cases in France. J Anim Physiol Anim Nutr 2010;94:712–20.

31. Puschner B, Aleman M. Lead toxicosis in the horse: A review. Equine Vet Educ 2010;22:526–30.

32. Dyson S, Taylor P, Whitwell K. Femoral nerve paralysis after general anaesthesia. Equine Vet J 1988;20:376–80.

33. Bootes BW. A fatal paralysis in foals from Ixodes holocyclus Neumann infestation. Aust Vet J 1963;38:68–9.

34. Mirtschin PJ, Masci P, Paton DC, et al. Snake bites recorded by veterinary practices in Australia. Aust Vet J 1998;76:195–8.

35. Aleman M. A review of equine muscle disorders. Neuromuscul Disord 2008;18: 277–87.

36. Valberg SJ. Diseases of muscles. In: Smith BP, ed. Large Animal Internal Medicine. 4th ed. St. Louis: Mosby Elsevier, 2009;1388–418.

37. MacLeay JM. Disorders of the musculoskeletal system. In: Reed SM, Warwick MB, Sellon DC, editors. Equine internal medicine. 3rd edition. St Louis (MO): Saunders Elsevier; 2010. p. 488–544.

38. Jayawardane P, Senanayake N, Dawson A. Electrophysiological correlates of intermediate syndrome following acute organophophate poisoning. Clin Toxicol 2009; 47:193–205.

39. Lalli G, Bohnert S, Deinhardt K, et al. The journey of tetanus and botulinum neurotoxins in neurons. Trends Microbiol 2003;11:431–7.

40. Goonetilleke A, Harris JB. Clostridial neurotoxins. J Neurol Neurosurg 2004;75: 35–9.

41. Hegreberg GA, Reed SM. Skeletal muscle changes associated with equine myotonic dystrophy. Acta Neuropathol 1990;80:426–31.

42. Reed SM, Hegreberg GA, Bayly WM, et al. Progressive myotonia in foals resembling human dystrophia myotonica. Muscle Nerve 1988;11:291–6.

43. Montagna P, Liguori R, Monari L, et al. Equine muscular dystrophy with myotonia. Clin Neurophysiol 2001;112:294–9.

44. Jamison JM, Baird JD, Smith-Maxie LL, et al. A congenital form of myotonia with dystrophic changes in a Quarter horse. Equine Vet J 1987;19:353–8.

45. Madigan JE, Valberg SJ, Ragle C, et al. Muscle spasms associated with ear tick (Otobius megnini) infestations in five horses. J Am Vet Med Assoc 1995;207:74–6.

46. Lunn DP, Mayhew IG. The neurological evaluation of horses. Equine Vet Educ 1989;1:94–101.

47. Wijnberg ID, van der Kolk JH, Franssen H, et al. Electromyographic changes of motor unit activity in horses with induced hypocalcemia and hypomagnesemia. Am J Vet Res 2002;63:849–56.

48. Wang S, McDonnell EH, Sedor FA, et al. pH effects on measurements of ionized calcium and ionized magnesium in blood. Arch Pathol Lab Med 2002;126:947–50.
49. Dumitru D, Zwarts MJ. The electrodiagnostic medicine consultation: approach and report generation. In: Dumitru D, Amato AA, Zwarts MJ, editors. Electrodiagnostic medicine. 2nd edition. Philadelphia: Hanley & Belfus; 2002. p. 515–40.
50. Aminoff MJ. Clinical electromyography. In: Aminoff MJ, editor. Electrodiagnosis in clinical neurology. 4th edition. Philadelphia: Churchill Livingstone; 1999. p. 223–52.
51. Wijnberg ID, Back W, de Jong M, et al. The role of electromyography in clinical diagnosis of neuromuscular locomotor problems in the horse. Equine Vet J 2004; 36:718–22.
52. Wijnberg ID, Franssen H, Jansen GH, et al. Quantitative electromyographic examination in myogenic disorders of 6 horses. J Vet Intern Med 2003;17:185–93.
53. Wijnberg ID. A review of the use of electromyography (EMG) in equine neurological diseases. Equine Vet Educ 2005;17:123–7.
54. Wijnberg ID, van der Kolk JH, Franssen H, et al. Needle electromyography in the horse compared with its principles in man: a review. Equine Vet J 2003;35:9–17.
55. Wijnberg ID, Franssen H, van der Kolk JH, et al. Quantitative motor unit action potential analysis of skeletal muscles in the Warmblood horse. Equine Vet J 2002; 34:556–61.
56. Naylor JM, Nickel DD, Trimino G, et al. Hyperkalemic periodic paralysis in homozygous and heterozygous horses: a co-dominant genetic condition. Equine Vet J 1999;31:153–9.
57. Daube JR, Devon IR. Needle electromyography. Muscle Nerve 2009;39:244–70.
58. Aleman M, Watson JL, Williams DC, et al. Myopathy in horses with pituitary pars intermedia dysfunction (Cushing's disease). Neuromuscul Disord 2006;16:737–44.
59. Spier SJ, Carlson GP, Holliday TA, et al. Hyperkalemic periodic paralysis in horses. J Am Vet Med Assoc 1990;197:1009–17.
60. Daube JR. Nerve conduction studies. In: Aminoff MJ, editor. Electrodiagnosis in clinical neurology. 4th edition. Philadelphia: Churchill Livingstone; 1999. p. 253–89.
61. Anor S, Espadaler JM, Monreal L, et al. Electrically elicited blink reflex in horses with trigeminal and facial nerve blocks. Am J Vet Res 1999;60:1287–91.
62. Whalen LR, Wheeler DW, LeCouteur RA, et al. Sensory nerve conduction velocity of the caudal cutaneous sural and medial cutaneous antebrachial nerves of adult horses. Am J Vet Res 1994;55:892–7.
63. Wheeler SJ. Effect of age on sensory nerve conduction velocity in the horse. Res Vet Sci 1990;48:141–4.
64. Wheeler SJ. Influence of limb temperature on sensory nerve conduction velocity in horses. Am J Vet Res 1989;50:1817–9.
65. Zarucco L, Driessen B, Scandella M, et al. Sensory nerve conduction and nociception in the equine lower forelimb during perineural bupivacaine infusion along the palmar nerves. Can J Vet Res 2010;74:305–13.
66. Blythe LL, Kitchell RL, Holliday TA, et al. Sensory nerve conduction velocities in forelimb of ponies. Am J Vet Res 1983;44:1419–26.
67. Blythe LL, Engel HN, Rowe KE. Comparison of sensory nerve conduction velocities in horses versus ponies. Am J Vet Res 1988;49:2138–42.
68. Henry RW, Diesem CD. Proximal equine radial and median motor nerve conduction velocity. Am J Vet Res 1981;42:1819–22.
69. Henry RW, Diesem CD, Wiechers DO. Evaluation of equine radial and median nerve conduction velocities. Am J Vet Res 1979;40:1406–10.
70. Thomson RM, Parry GJ. Neuropathies associated with excessive exposure to lead. Muscle Nerve 2006;33:732–41.

71. Cuddon PA. Electrophysiology in neuromuscular disease. Vet Clin North Am Small Anim Pract 2002;32:31–62.
72. Aleman M, Williams DC, Nieto JE, et al. Repetitive stimulation of the common peroneal nerve as a diagnostic aid for botulism in foals. J Vet Intern Med 2011;25: 365–72.
73. Schaeppi U, Teste M, Siegenthaler U. Single fiber electromyography. A method for the evaluation of motor axonopathy during toxicity studies in dogs. Agents Actions 1981;11:510–4.
74. Anor S, Lipsitz D, Williams DC, et al. Evaluation of jitter by stimulated single-fiber electromyography in normal dogs. J Vet Intern Med 2003;17:545–50.
75. Wijnberg ID, Sleutjens J, Van der Kolk JH, et al. Effect of head and neck position on outcome of quantitative neuromuscular diagnostic techniques in Warmblood riding horses directly following moderate exercise. Equine Vet J 2010;42:S261–7.
76. Dickinson PJ, LeCouteur RA. Muscle and nerve biopsy. Vet Clin North Am Small Anim Pract 2002;32:63–102.
77. Rhee HS, Steel CM, Derksen FJ, et al. Immunohistochemical analysis of laryngeal muscles in normal horses and horses with subclinical recurrent laryngeal neuropathy. J Histochem Cytochem 2009;57:787–800.
78. Matiasek K, Gais P, Rodenacker K, et al. Stereological characteristics of the equine accessory nerve. Anat Histol Embryol 2008;37:205–13.
79. Maher O, Davis DM, Drake C, et al. Pull-through technique for palmar digital neurectomy: forty-one horses (1998–2004). Vet Surg 2007;37:87–93.
80. Jackman BR, Baxter GM, Doran RE, et al. Palmar digital neurectomy in horses: 57 cases (1984–1990). Vet Surg 1993;22:285–8.
81. Williams JW, Pascoe JR, Meagher DM, et al. Effects of left recurrent laryngeal neurectomy, prosthetic laryngoplasty, and subtotal arytenoidectomy on upper airway pressure during maximal exertion. Vet Surg 1990;19:136–41.
82. Jackson CA, de Lahunta A, Cummings JF, et al. Spinal accessory nerve biopsy as an antemortem diagnostic test for equine motor neuron disease. Equine Vet J 1996; 28:215–20.
83. Wheeler SJ. Quantitative and qualitative morphology of equine peripheral nerve: teased fibre studies. Res Vet Sci 1990;48:145–51.
84. Alexander K, Dobson H. Ultrasonography of peripheral nerves in the normal adult horse. Vet Radiol Ultrasound 2003;44:456–64.
85. Khan J, Harrison TB, Rich MM. Mechanisms of neuromuscular dysfunction in critical illness. Crit Care Clin 2008;24:165–75.
86. Stevens RD, Marshall SA, Cornblath DR, et al. A framework for diagnosing and classifying intensive care unit-acquired weakness. Crit Care Med 2009;37:S309–15.
87. Toribio RE, Kohn CW, Hardy J, et al. Alterations in serum parathyroid hormone and electrolyte concentrations and urinary excretion of electrolytes in horses with induced endotoxemia. J Vet Intern Med 2005;19:223–31.
88. Toribio RE, Kohn CW, Chew DJ, et al. Comparison of serum parathyroid hormone and ionized calcium and magnesium concentratios and fractional urinary clearance of calcium and phosphorus in healty horses and horses with enterocolitis. Am J Vet Res 2001;62:938–47.
89. Hurcombe SD, Toribio RE, Slovis NM, et al. Calcium regulating hormones and serum calcium and magnesium concentrations in septic and critically ill foals and their association with survival. J Vet Intern Med 2009;32:335–43.
90. Yvorchuk-St JK. Neuritis of the cauda equina. Vet Clin North Am Equine Pract 1987;3:421–7.

91. Wright JA, Fordyce PS, Edington N. Neuritis of the cauda equina in the horse. J Comp Pathol 1987;97:667–75.
92. Greenwood AG, Baker J, McLeish I. Neuritis of the cauda equina in a horse. Equine Vet J 1973;5:111–5.
93. Cummings JF, de Lahunta A, Timoney JF. Neuritis of the cauda equina, a chronic idiopathic polyradiculoneuritis in the horse. Acta Neuropathol 1979;46:17–24.
94. van Galen G, Cassart D, Sandersen C, et al. The composition of the inflammatory infiltrate in three cases of polyneuritis equi. Equine Vet J 2008;40:185–8.
95. Rousseaux CG, Futcher KG, Clark EG, et al. Cauda equina neuritis: a chronic idiopathic polyneuritis in two horses. Can Vet J 1984;25:214–8.
96. Rimaila-Parnanen E. Neuritis of the cauda equina in a horse. Nord Vet Med 1976; 28:464–7.
97. Manning JP, Gosser HS. Neuritis of the cauda equina in horses. Vet Med Small Anim Clin 1973;68:1162–5.
98. Billinski J, Sprinkle T, Lee J. A case of cauda equina neuritis. Vet Med Small Anim Clin 1977;72:597–8.
99. Scarratt WK, Jortner BS. Neuritis of the cauda equina in a yearling filly. Compend Contin Educ Pract 1985;7:S197–202.
100. Vatistas N, Mayhew IG, Whitwell KE, et al. Polyneuritis equi: a clinical review incorporating a case report of a horse displaying unconventional signs. Progress Vet Neurol 1991;2:67–72.
101. Hahn CN. Polyneuritis equi: the role of T-lymphocytes and importance of differential clinical signs. Equine Vet J 2008;40:100.
102. Kadlubowski M, Ingram PL. Circulating antibodies to the neuritogenic myelin protein, P2, in neuritis of the cauda equina of the horse. Nature 1981;293:299–300.
103. Klingeborn B, Dinter Z, Hughes RA. Antibody to neuritogenic myelin protein P2 in equine paresis due to equine herpesvirus 1. Zentralbl Veterinarmed B 1983;30: 137–40.
104. Maselli RA, Bakshi N. Botulism. Muscle Nerve 2000;23:1137–44.
105. Whitlock RH. Botulism, type C: Experimental and field cases in horses. Equine Pract 1996;18:11–7.
106. Gudmundsson SH. Type B botulinum intoxication in horses: case report and literature review. Equine Vet Educ 1997;9:156–9.
107. Schoenbaum MA, Hall SM, Glock RD, et al. An outbreak of type C botulinum in 12 horses and a mule. J Am Vet Med Assoc 2000;217:365–8.
108. Wilkins PA, Palmer JE. Botulism in foals less than 6 months of age: 30 cases (1989–2002). J Vet Intern Med 2003;17:702–7.
109. Johnson AL, McAdams SC, Whitlock RH. Type A botulism in horses in the United States: a review of the past ten years (1998–2008). J Vet Diagn Invest 2010;22: 165–73.
110. Galey FD. Botulism in the horse. Vet Clin North Am Equine Pract 2001;17:579–88.
111. Kinde H, Bettey RL, Ardans A, et al. Clostridium botulinum type-C intoxication associated with consumption of processed alfalfa hay cubes in horses. J Am Vet Med Assoc 1991;199:742–6.
112. Steinman A, Kachtan I, Levi O, et al. Seroprevalence of antibotulinum neurotoxin type C antibodies in horses in Israel. Equine Vet J 2007;39:232–5.
113. Gerber v, Straub R, Frey J. Equine botulism and acute pasture myodystrophy: new soil-borne emerging diseases in Switzerland? Schweiz Arch Tierheilkd 2006;148: 553–9.
114. Grumelli C, Verderio C, Pozzi D, et al. Internalization and mechanism of action of clostridial toxins in neurons. Neurotoxicology 2005;26:761–7.

115. Comella CL, Pullman SL. Botulinum toxins in neurological disease. Muscle Nerve 2004;29:628–44.

116. Catsicas S, Grenningloh G, Pich EM. Nerve-terminal proteins: to fuse to learn. Trends Neurosci 1994;17:368–73.

117. Newton JR, Wylie CE, Proudman CJ, et al. Equine grass sickness: Are we any nearer to answers on cause and prevention after a century of research? Equine Vet J 2010;42:477–81.

118. Adam-Castrillo D, White NAn, Donaldson LL, et al. Effects of injection of botulinum toxin type B into the external anal sphincter on anal pressure of horses. Am J Vet Res 2004;65:26–30.

119. Lindberg A, Skarin H, Knutsson R, et al. Real-time PCR for Clostridium botulinum type C neurotoxin (BoNTC) gene, also covering a chimeric C/D sequence-application on outbreaks of botulism in poultry. Vet Microbiol 2010;146:118–23.

120. Umeda K, Seto Y, Kohda T, et al. A novel multiplex PCR method for Clostridium botulinum neurotoxin type A gene cluster typing. Microbiol Immunol 2010;54:308–12.

121. Stahl C, Unger L, Mazuet C, et al. Immune response of horses to vaccination with the recombinant Hc domain of botulinum neurotoxin types C and D. Vaccine 2009;27:5661–6.

122. Frey J, Eberle S, Stahl C, et al. Alternative vaccination against equine botulism (BoNT/C). Equine Vet J 2007;39:516–20.

123. Kay G, Knottenbelt DC. Tetanus in equids: A report of 56 cases. Equine Vet Educ 2007;19:107–12.

124. Toribio RE, Kohn CW, Rourke KM, et al. Effects of hypercalcemia on serum concentrations of magnesium, potassium, and phosphate and urinary excretion of electrolytes in horses. Am J Vet Res 2007;68:543–54.

125. Johansson AM, Gardner SY, Jones SL, et al. Hypomagnesemia in hospitalized horses. J Vet Intern Med 2003;17:860–7.

126. De Bleeker J. The intermediate syndrome in organophosphate poisoning: an overview of experimental and clinical observations. Clin Toxicol 1995;33:683–6.

127. Karanth S, Pope C. In vitro inhibition of blood cholinesterase activities from horse, cow and rat by tetrachlorvinphos. Int J Toxicol 2003;22:429–33.

128. Karalliedde L, Henry J. Effects of organophosphates on skeletal muscle. Hum Exp Toxicol 1993;12:289–96.

129. Hunt LM, Valberg SJ, Steffenhagen K, et al. An epidemiological study of myopathies in Warmblood horses. Equine Vet J 2008;40:171–7.

130. Firshman AM, Baird JD, Valberg SJ. Prevalences and clinical signs of polysaccharide storage myopathy and shivers in Belgian draft horses. J Am Vet Med Assoc 2005;227:1958–64.

Toxins and Adverse Drug Reactions Affecting the Equine Nervous System

Dominic R. Dawson, DVM

KEYWORDS

• Adverse drug reaction • Toxic • Equine • Neurologic

This article provides an overview of the more common toxins and adverse drug reactions, along with more rare toxins and reactions that result in neurologic dysfunction in horses.

BOTULISM

Botulism is caused by exposure to botulinum neurotoxin produced by *Clostridium botulinum*, a spore-forming, anaerobic, Gram-positive bacterium. All 8 botulinum toxins inhibit the release of acetylcholine by disrupting various stages of synaptic vesicle docking and fusion.[1] Horses typically develop botulism in 3 ways: (1) ingestion of preformed toxin via contaminated forage, grain, or water source; (2) elaboration of the toxin in the gastrointestinal tract, of foals mainly, after ingestion and spore germination; or (3) wound contamination with spores leading to germination and toxin production. There are 8 different serotypes, differentiated by their toxins; Types A, B, and C are the most commonly reported causes of botulism in horses in North America. There is preliminary evidence that *C botulinum* Type C may be involved with the emerging grass sickness syndrome (EGS), a polyneuropathy seen in Europe.[2] The types can vary with respect to clinical signs,[3–5] geographical distribution,[6,7] and most common route of exposure.[4–7] Type A may be more common west of the Mississippi, while Type B seems more problematic on the East Coast (often associated with ingestion of moldy forages); however, clinical signs appear similar.[6] In foals, toxicoinfectious botulism with Type B is more frequent.[7] With Type C, the source of contamination is carrion versus moldy hay[4] and dysphagia is variable.[3–5]

Clinical signs with all types include progressive symmetrical flaccid paresis; weak anal, tail, tongue, and eyelid tone; dysphagia; slow pupillary light reflexes; mydriasis; respiratory distress; and death.[5,6,8,9] Horses generally do not exhibit conscious proprioceptive deficits and remain responsive, which helps differentiate botulism from

The author has nothing to disclose.

William Pritchard Veterinary Medical Teaching Hospital, University of California, Davis, One Garrod Avenue, Davis, CA 95616, USA

E-mail address: drdawson@ucdavis.edu

other neurologic diseases with weakness and recumbency. While severity of signs is presumably dose-related, Type A may have higher case fatality rates.[6] In addition to signs directly related to the neurotoxin, horses can experience ocular and musculo-skeletal trauma from struggling to rise.

The mouse bioassay[a] using feces or gastric contents remains the gold standard of diagnosis; however, results can require considerable time. Future testing directions include an enzyme-linked immunosorbent assay and endopeptidase assays[10] and polymerase chain reaction testing.[11] Forage, grain, feces, gastrointestinal contents, water source, and wound swabs can all be tested; however, confirmation is difficult and diagnosis is often made on history and clinical signs alone.

Treatment should focus on neutralizing any unbound toxin with antitoxin and supporting the patient's vital functions. Many affected horses can be supported via regular nasogastric tube administrations of gruel feedings and water. Horses recalcitrant to intubation and very severely affected horses may require intravenous fluids, partial or total parenteral nutrition, and ventilatory and circulatory support until remodeling of muscle endplates occurs, which can be up to 1 month. Antitoxin is only effective against unbound botulinum toxin and early administration is crucial. Patients may deteriorate further after administration due to toxin already bound to receptors. Currently, polyvalent[a,b] and Type B monovalent[c] antitoxins are available, but there is a substantial difference in price. On the West Coast, if financially feasible, the polyvalent is recommended as it contains antibodies against both A and C.[6] A new antitoxin containing $F(ab)_2$ against Type A has effectively treated botulism with fewer side effects in mice.[12] In foals, mechanical ventilation greatly improves outcome,[8,9] and frequent monitoring of arterial blood gases in the first 36 to 48 hours of exposure helps identify cases requiring ventilation.[9] Antibiotics are not routine in human toxicoinfectious botulism due to the concern for increased toxin release following vegetative cell death and lysis.[13] However, if secondary complications arise necessitating antibiotics such as aspiration pneumonia or severe pressure sores, then care should be taken to avoid antimicrobials that potentiate neuromuscular blockade such as aminoglycosides and tetracycline.[8,14] Weak horses may suffer life-threatening muscle tears or fractures when allowed to rise on their own without sling support (author, personal observation); however, slung horses require observation for respiratory difficulty due to thoracic compression and weakened respiratory muscular effort.

In recumbent horses, the case fatality is high, but foal survival rates can reach 96%,[9] likely due to feasibility of mechanical ventilation and better management of recumbent cases. Better detection of the early, subtle clinical signs in human botulism cases may explain improved outcomes compared to horses.[15] Monitoring of exposed horses' tongue tone and performance of grain tests (normal horses can eat 8 oz of sweet feed in under 2 minutes) may similarly improve outcomes.

Vaccination is thought to be protective in adult horses[16,17]; however, passive transfer of antibodies from vaccinated dams significantly reduces, but may not eliminate, botulism in foals.[9] Worldwide, 2 vaccines are available[d,e]; however, in the United States only vaccination against Type B is available.[c] Vaccination studies demonstrate lack of cross-protection between types[17]; therefore, horses on the

---

[a]Botulism polyvalent antitoxin, Botulism Laboratory, New Bolton Center, Kennett Square, PA.
[b]Lake Immunogenics Inc, Ontario, NY.
[c]Monovalent antitoxin against Type B, PLasvacc USA Inc, Templeton, CA.
[d]Neogen Corporation, Lexington, Kentucky, USA.
[e]Onderstepoort Biological Products, Onderstepoort, South Africa.

West Coast are likely at risk for Types A and C, despite vaccination against Type B. Newer vaccines against Types C and D using recombinant technology are currently being studied in horses[16,17] both for botulism and possibly against EGS.[2] Horses recovering from botulism should still be vaccinated because protection from antitoxin administration is transient and the exposure dose required to cause significant clinical disease is still too low to promote protective immunoglobulin production.

While vaccination may play an important role in prevention and is recommended in regions with a high occurance of Type B botulism, preventing exposure to the toxin is vital. Limiting environments conducive to *C. botulinum* sporulation reduces the risk for ingestion of preformed toxin. Recommendations include appropriate storage of feed to prevent moisture and spoiling, along with inspection and disposal of any wet or spoiled feed. In one outbreak, exposure occurred from spoiled hay allowed to accumulate around the feeder.[6] Haylage, round hay bales, and silage should be used with caution and appropriately acidic pH and storage requirements observed. Outbreaks with milled feeds[4] and from birds carrying contaminated material from improperly buried carcasses up to 3 miles away[5] have been reported. Additionally, a horse injected intramuscularly with 2500 U of botulinum toxin Type B experienced systemic botulism[18]; therefore, the practice of injecting botulinum toxins cannot be recommended for asthetic use alone. Caution should be exercised when using botulinum toxins for therapeutic purposes (eg, treatment of stringhalt or laminitis) due to the possibility of iatrogenic botulism.

ADVERSE INJECTION REACTIONS (PROCAINE, VENOUS AIR EMBOLISM, INTRACAROTID INJECTION)

Procaine, a depot salt usually administered intramuscularly with benzylpenicillin, allows for longer therapeutic antimicrobial concentrations. Normally procaine is slowly absorbed and plasma esterase hydrolyzes it to the nontoxic *para*-aminobenzoic acid (PABA). However, a sudden large bolus can overwhelm the plasma esterase, leading to violent and sometimes deadly reactions. Humans report anxiety and hallucinations with intravenous procaine.[19] Clinical signs in horses are similar and include startled behavior, sudden rearing or violent circling, ataxia, muscle tremors, vocalization, seizures, nystagmus, sweating, transient blindness, collapse, and death.[20–22] While not entirely known, procaine is proposed to exert its effect directly on the central nervous system (CNS) and resolution of signs can occur anywhere from a few minutes to up to 2 weeks after the acute reaction.[22] These unpredictable, usually immediate, reactions can occur upon first administration or after multiple uneventful doses, and after appropriate dose and injection technique, making avoidance difficult. Interestingly, new work shows a possible link between decreased plasma esterase levels and procaine benzylpenicillin reactions, along with possible genetic differences in procaine sensitivity.[22] Reactions may be more frequent after multiple intramuscular injections either due to increased vascularization of injected muscle[21] or possibly due to "kindling," an increased response after repetitive stimulation over time of a subthreshold stimuli.[23] Horses experiencing an acute reaction should be safely contained as self-trauma can be life threatening. Immediate treatment is often impossible; however, the majority of horses' clinical signs resolve without specific treatment. If possible, further use of procaine-containing products should be avoided, but if no other antimicrobial options exist, continued use is possible.[22]

Venous air emboli may occur more often than realized as horses can handle up to 0.25 mL/kg of air intravenously before exhibiting signs.[24] Typically, any venous air passes into the pulmonary circulation, diffuses into the alveolus, and is expelled with expiration. However, high volumes of venous air can prevent blood from reaching the right heart and the pulmonary circulation because air remains trapped in either the right atrium or ventricle and forms an air lock. Signs may be due to cerebral hypoxemia and ischemia[25] and include labored breathing, tachypnea, ataxia, weakness, and collapse.[25,26] Pruritis is a common finding in humans[27] and has been reported in horses secondary to venous air embolism.[28] Neurologic signs can be delayed up to 18 hours, persist for up to 3 weeks, and include nystagmus, proprioceptive deficits, and head pressing.[25] If a venous air embolism is suspected, then administering high doses of intravenous fluids along with oxygen insufflation or performing intermittent positive pressure ventilation under general anesthesia may help alleviate signs.[28] Removal of air via "vacuuming" with central venous access has been performed in severely affected humans but has not been reported in horses.[28] If cerebral edema is suspected, then hypertonic saline, mannitol, and antioxidant and anti-inflammatory therapies such as flunixin meglumine, vitamin C, vitamin E, thiamine, or DMSO may be beneficial.[25] Prevention involves careful monitoring of extension sets, catheter injection ports, and fluid lines. Some authors recommend placing jugular catheters "upward" in the vein; however, this carries a higher risk for thrombophlebitis and clotting.[28]

Intracarotid injections can cause a variety of signs ranging from short-term collapse to significant cerebral necrosis and death. Consequences of the injection vary depending on the dose and type of drug. Drugs crossing the blood-brain barrier (BBB) cause edema, hemorrhage, neuronal necrosis, vascular necrosis, and thrombosis[29] most commonly of the cerebrum and thalamus on the ipsilateral side of injection.[30] Clinical signs include muscle tremors, stertorous respiration, pupillary dilation, collapse, seizures, and death[31] and can be delayed as in one case with persistent blindness and left laryngeal hemiplegia 4 days after intracarotid injection of phenylbutazone.[32] In one experiment, promazine, acepromazine, thiopental, magnesium sulfate, and calcium gluconate induced clinical signs after intracarotid injection.[29] Importantly, not all horses reacted when given these drugs intra-arterially, showing that some individual difference is present.[29] However, anecdotal reports of adverse reactions after intracarotid injections for multiple other drugs, including alpha-2 agonists and phenylbutazone, exist. Treatment is supportive and symptomatic. Careful observation for a few days should be performed as clinical signs can be delayed.

LONG-TERM SEDATIVES (RESERPINE AND FLUPHENAZINE)

Reserpine, an indole alkaloid, is used for long-term sedation and treatment of agalactia in mares exposed to fescue, despite lack of approval for equine use. Obtained from the root of *Rauwolfia serpentine*, reserpine exerts its effect via long-term depletion of catecholamine and serotonin stores in organs and reduction of catecholamine uptake by sympathetic neurons.[33] Therefore, adverse effects are related to diminished sympathetic tone and adrenergic inhibition[33] and possibly also direct oxidative damage.[34] Clinical signs of intoxication in horses include agitation, hyperexcitability, muscle fasciculation, bradycardia, miosis, ptosis, whole body sweating, nasal edema, priapism, diarrhea, and abdominal discomfort.[35,36] Reserpine can be detected in the blood, but not urine, but rapid clearance after single doses makes confirmation difficult. If repeated doses are given plasma levels may remain detectable for up to 48 hours.[37] Studies looking at dosage for reserpine have suggested 1 mg/450 kg parenterally; total doses of 5 to 10 mg have caused colic, sweating, flatulence, miosis, ptosis, and depression.[38] Although there is no specific antidote, treatment consists of supportive care, reducing stimulation, and management of the penile prolapse, although there is evidence that vitamin C and vitamin E have beneficial effects. As significant nasal edema can develop, monitoring of airway patency is recommended. Improvement may be seen after 48 hours, with full resolution expected by 4 to 5 days.[36]

Another frequently used long-term sedative, fluphenazine (decanoate or enanthate), can cause extrapyramidal effects in horses. There are limited pharmacokinetic studies of fluphenazine and horses may be more sensitive to adverse effects due to a more extensive extrapyramidal system.[39,40] Other animals appears to have a genetic predisposition to adverse effects; however, this is unstudied in horses.[41] Fluphenazine blocks dopamine[42] and clinical signs involve intermittent compulsive circling, repetitive and often extreme head and neck movements, pawing, severe agitation with intermittent obtundation, flank-biting, profuse sweating, hypermetria, buckling of the forelimbs, and coarse muscular tremors.[39,40,42] Clinical signs can occur after single or multiple doses and within 16 to 72 hours after drug administration.[39,40,42] Reported doses leading to toxicity vary from 25 mg to 125 mg intramuscularly; however, a single 40-mg dose given intravenously resulted in clinical signs that necessitated euthanasia of the horse approximately 3 days later.[39,40,42] Intravenous administration may represent a higher risk as the aforementioned horse had lower plasma fluphenazine concentrations than surviving horses. Diagnosis involves history of fluphenazine administration, clinical signs, and detection in the blood via high-pressure liquid chromatography.[40] Clinical pathologic changes are nonspecific, and in one case cerebrospinal fluid (CSF) was unremarkable.[42] In one report, the following treatments were attempted with no improvement: butorphanol tartrate, diazepam, dimethyl sulfoxide (DMSO), morphine, detomidine hydrochloride, romifidine, and chloral hydrate.[39] Administration of diphenhydramine hydrochloride can have variable success[39,40,42]; however, consistent improvement has been seen with sodium pentobarbital (2 mg/kg IV as repeated boluses or as CRI over 120 minutes).[39,40] Success was also seen with benztropine mesylate (0.018–0.035 mg/kg po q 12 h).[39] One important secondary complication is nasal and head edema due to either self-trauma or abnormal head position with heavy sedation. In one case respiratory distress occurred, necessitating an emergency tracheostomy.[39] Anti-inflammatories for muscle trauma and oral laxatives to assist with ileus caused by prolonged sedation may be indicated.[40] Improvement is gradual and horses may continue to show clinical signs for up to 9 days,[39] necessitating repeated sedation and treatment. Thus far, no long-term effects have been reported. Prevention involves judicious use of long-term sedatives. Fluphenazine can be excreted in milk, so foals whose dams receive fluphenazine should be monitored.[43]

IVERMECTIN

Ivermectin toxicity has previously been reported usually after overdoses[44]; however, 3 horses recently experienced ataxia, hypersensitivity, bilateral mydriasis, head pressing, apparent blindness, decreased pupillary light reflexes, lack of menace response, hypersalivation, and decreased lip tone approximately 18 to 24 hours after receiving an appropriate oral dose of ivermectin paste.[45] The 2 surviving horses exhibited clinical signs for up to 9 days but were clinically unremarkable 6 months later. Previous reports described impaired vision, ataxia, and depression after horses received 2.0 mg/kg po for 2 consecutive days.[46] By potentiating the release of the inhibitory neurotransmitter GABA, ivermectin causes chloride ion influx, which hyperpolarizes neuronal cells, leading to flaccid paralysis in invertebrates.[47] Unlike invertebrates with GABA receptors in the peripheral nervous system, mammals only have GABA receptors in the CNS and an intact BBB prevents adverse effects. Exposure to silverleaf nightshade (*Solanum eleagnifolium*), which can be found in many southern states, was suspected to cause breakdown of the BBB and subsequent ivermectin toxicosis in 8 of 14 horses.[48] Diagnosis must be made on history of exposure, as serum levels are not conclusive for toxicosis. Upon post-mortem, brain tissue concentrations of ivermectin greater than 4 μg/kg may confirm ivermectin toxicosis as in a normal animal, the BBB should restrict ivermectin concentrations in the CNS.[49] Specific antidotes are lacking for avermectin toxicosis and treatment is supportive. Reported treatments include flunixin meglumine, diazepam, detomidine hydrochloride, and/or dexamethasone along with nursing care and intravenous fluid therapy.[45] Corticosteroids may or may not be of benefit, as inflammation may not contribute to clinical signs. Fluids do not increase excretion as ivermectin is excreted in the feces. Other, unproved, treatments in horses include neostigmine and sarmazenil, a competitive GABA receptor antagonist used in a foal with moxidectin overdose.[50] Recently, intravenous lipid administration proved to be an effective therapy for moxidectin toxicity in a dog.[51] Moxidectin should not be given in foals under 4 months of age.

IONOPHORES (MONENSIN, SALINOMYCIN, AND LASALOCID)

While commonly used in food animals, horses are highly sensitive to ionophore antibiotics and intoxications are frequently life threatening.[52,53] Ionophores increase membrane permeability causing abnormal ion fluxes.[54] Clinical signs include colic, lethargy, anorexia, restlessness, recumbency, respiratory distress, myositis, cardiomyopathy, sweating, and death.[52,53] While the more dramatic clinical signs tend to be related to the skeletal and cardiac muscles, horses can experience damage to neurologic tissues that manifest in ataxia, paresis, and muscle atrophy.[52,53,55] In some cases, ataxia and seizures may be the only sign seen.[52] Widespread peripheral nerve swelling with degeneration of axons and myelin sheaths was seen in the peripheral nervous system with salinomycin toxicosis.[56] In contrast, monensin-induced ataxic horses have had minimal to no histopathologic changes in the neural tissues.[52,55] Clinical signs of toxicosis typically develop within a few days of exposure and, depending on the dose, symptoms can vary from sudden death to chronic mild changes. Diagnosis is often based on clinical signs, history of exposure, and histopathologic findings. Detection of ionophores can be difficult due to limited tissue accumulation; however, feed; stomach contents; liver, heart, or skeletal muscle; and stomach tissues can be tested. Reports of LD_{50} for ionophores include 0.6 (salinomycin), 2 to 3 (monensin), and 15 to 21.5 (lasalocid) mg/kg.[57,58] Lab findings typical of ionophore toxicity include myoglobinuria, increased serum activities of creatine kinase, aspartate aminotransferase, alkaline phosphatase, and lactate dehydrogenase.[53,59] In addition, some horses exhibit hyponatremia, hypochloremia, hypocalcemia, hypomagnesemia, severe hyperglycemia, and evidence of hypovolemia.[52] Elevated cardiac troponin I levels at 24 to 72 hours postexposure should prompt intervention with vitamin E, selenium, and supportive care, and horses with severely elevated levels by 48 hours are at higher risk for significant disease.[55] CSF analysis in one case was unremarkable.[53] Care should be taken to avoid drugs that potentiate ionophore's effects: chloramphenicol, tiamulin, erythromycin, sulfonamides, triacetyloleandromycin, and cardiac glycosides. Currently no specific treatment exists; however, administration of vitamin E and selenium may help prevent cell injury.[60] If provided early enough, gastric lavage and charcoal can decrease concentrations of absorbable ionophores. Animals can die suddenly from minor stress due to worsened ionic flux, and therefore only necessary interventions should be performed. Even with appropriate intervention, prognosis is poor. Ataxia after salinomycin toxicity can persist for months, along with muscle atrophy and decreased athletic performance.[53] Long-term cardiac monitoring is encouraged as cardiac disease can be delayed[52] and/or persistent.[55]

MAGNESIUM SULFATE

While generally a safe oral laxative, intoxications with magnesium sulfate occur after iatrogenic overdose, increased intestinal absorption due to mucosal compromise or delayed transit time,[61] or decreased systemic clearance of magnesium by the kidney. Magnesium depresses the CNS and neuromuscular junction by inhibiting acetylcholine release. Excesses can cause muscle tremors, flaccid paralysis, depressed reflexes, CNS depression, tachycardia, paralytic ileus, and respiratory distress as early as 4 hours after administration.[61,62] Diagnosis is based on serum magnesium levels with early clinical signs seen at concentrations of 3 to 5 mg/dL.[63] Once toxicosis has occurred, any magnesium-containing fluids or oral treatments should be discontinued. Unfortunately, charcoal does not bind magnesium; however, calcium antagonizes the effects of magnesium at the neuromuscular junction. Therefore, intravenous calcium supplementation should be initiated immediately (250 mL of 23% calcium gluconate diluted in 1 L saline) and repeated as necessary.[61] Diuresis with magnesium-free fluids will promote excretion, and if renal function is adequate, furosemide may be added. Aminoglycosides should be avoided as they potentiate neuromuscular blockade.[64] One indicator of early hypermagnesemia in humans is loss of the patellar reflexes, and this should be monitored in foals undergoing magnesium sulfate treatment. Additional monitoring of blood electrolytes, calcium, phosphorus, renal function, fluid intake and outputs, and ECG is indicated. Prevention centers on judicious oral and parenteral magnesium use, especially in horses with concurrent administration of potential gastrointestinal irritants such as dioctyl sodium sulfosuccinate,[61] decreased urinary output, severe ileus as increased transit time promotes excessive absorption,[65] or parathyroid compromise as parathyroid hormone promotes magnesium renal excretion.[66]

PROPYLENE GLYCOL

Nasogastric propylene glycol administration has occurred when mistaken for mineral oil.[67–69] Clinical signs can occur within minutes[67,69] due to severe metabolic acidosis secondary to increased D-lactate levels, leading to death within 24 hours.[67] Horses exhibit CNS depression, ataxia, salivation, sweating, abnormal breath odor, seizures, and colic.[67–69] Diagnosis is via history of exposure and detection of propylene glycol in renal tissue, blood, and urine.[67] In addition, Heinz bodies can develop post-intoxication.[67] Immediate intervention with stomach lavage, charcoal and mineral oil administration, fluid support, isotonic bicarbonate, and supportive care in addition to careful blood gas monitoring may prevent death.[68,69]

EQUINE LEUKOENCEPHALOMALACIA (MOLDY CORN INTOXICATION)

Equine leukoencephalomalacia occurs after exposure to fumonisin B_1 or B_2[70] mycotoxins produced by *Fusarium* fungal species that commonly contaminate cereal grains, especially corn. In a dose-dependent manner,[71] fumonisin B_1 inhibits sphingolipid biosynthesis theoretically leading to accumulation of sphingolipid intermediates and depletion of sphingolipid, an integral part of cell membrane function.[72,73] Interestingly, recent work showed unchanged brain sphingolipid levels after fumonisin B_1 exposure and instead suggests that accumulation of sphingolipid intermediates affects autoregulation of cerebral vascular beds leading to increased cerebral pressure and edema.[71] Regardless of mechanism, liquefactive necrosis of subcortical white matter ultimately develops. Subtle, early signs such as paralysis of the tongue and mild conscious proprioceptive deficits may be missed[71] and with continued exposure horses progress to often permanent hyperexcitability, aimless circling, head pressing, paresis, ataxia, blindness, quadriceps muscle atrophy, increased liver enzymes, and depression.[74] Fumonisin toxins also affect the liver and heart causing additional clinical signs. CSF analysis can reveal increased protein, albumin, albumin quotients, and IgG concentrations.[71] Morbidity and mortality are high with death sometimes occurring before clinical signs. However, early removal of contaminated feed and supportive treatment may improve outcome.[71] Fumonisin B_1 can be detected in feed and levels of 0.05 mg/kg body weight or greater are considered toxic.[71] Increased serum sphinganine and sphingosine concentrations may aid early diagnsis.[73] Treatment recommendations include anti-inflammatory and antiedema medications such as DMSO, glucocorticosteroids, or diuretics such as mannitol, along with calcium gluconate infusions (0.2 mg/kg/min) to improve cardiac output.[75,76] Adults, who have longer necks, are more prone to neurologic disease after exposure than are foals, possibly due to sphingosine-mediated decreased control of cerebral blood flow when the head is lowered.[71] If this is true, then affected horses may benefit from elevation of feed. Feed companies that screen their products for fumonisin should be used if possible.

EQUINE REFLEX HYPERTONIA (STRINGHALT)

Equine reflex hypertonia (ERH) is a symptom, not a diagnosis, typically classified into 2 different forms: idiopathic (also known as classic or spontaneous) ERH and acquired or Australian ERH associated with ingestion of *Hypochaeris radicata* (Australian dandelion), *Taraxacum officinale* (European dandelion), or *Malva parviflora* (mallow). Acquired ERH involves distal axonopathy of the longest myelinated nerves.[77,78] While most intoxications occur in the late summer and autumn when there is poor pasture quality, disease has been reproduced experimentally in the winter.[79,80] There appears to be significant variations in the toxicity of individual *H. radicata* with some plants not inducing the disease[79] and not all exposed horses exhibiting signs.[78] The etiology of the plants' toxicities is unknown at this time and they have a wide distribution throughout the United States. Horses with dandelion-acquired ERH have an unmistakable sudden and involuntary hyperflexion of one or both hindlimbs that can progress to recumbency.[78,80] The early signs of slight hyperflexion with backing or mild laryngeal dysfunction may be missed.[78] Differentiating classic from dandelion-acquired ERH can be difficult; however, the classic form is often unilateral, can be seen after injury, and is usually progressive over years, whereas the dandelion-acquired form can occur bilaterally, often has an acute onset as soon as 15 to 19 days after exposure,[78,79] and can be part of an outbreak.[81] In addition to the hindlimb abnormalities, horses can also experience forelimb involvement, muscle atrophy,[80] decreased panniculus reflex,[79] recurrent laryngeal dysfunction,[78] and behavioral changes including stupor, depression, and increased aggression.[78] Diagnosis of the dandelion-acquired form is based on a history of exposure, clinical signs, electromyography demonstrating dysfunction of the long digital extensor muscle and/or unusually large motor units, decreased nerve conduction velocity, or post-mortem examination.[78,82] A recent case was diagnosed ante-mortem via biopsies of the long digital extensor muscle and superficial peroneal nerve.[81] Once diagnosed, affected horses should be removed from contaminated pastures. Administration of CNS myorelaxants and tranquilizers such as phenytoin or acepromazine has improved clinical signs.[78,83] Treatment with anti-inflammatory drugs, DMSO, and vitamin E have been used; however, it is unknown if these specifically improved outcome or if removal of plant and rest were sufficient.[78] In refractory cases, myotenectomy of the lateral digital extensor tendon may help.[78] There are reported benefits in behavioral abnormalities but not gait abnormalities with taurine (10 mg po q 24 hours).[78] Horses typically recover over weeks to months once removed from the pasture,[79,81,83] but some require years[78,83] and laryngeal paralysis may persist even after gait normalization.[83] Pasture management to prevent dry, overgrazed pastures may decrease cases.[78]

OXYTROPIS (LOCOWEED) AND ASTRAGALUS spp.

Intoxication with plants or fungi producing swainsonine, a phytotoxin, is the most widespread poisonous plant problem for livestock in the western United States.[84] Plants from the genera *Oxytropis* (locoweed) and *Astragalus* (milkvetch) cause symptoms after considerable cumulative ingestion. Embellisia, a fungus isolated from *Oxytropic lambertii*, and *Rhizoctonia leguminicola*, a fungus infecting red clover, can also produce swainsonine. Swainsonine inhibits the lysosomal enzyme alpha-mannosidase,[85] causing abnormal substrate accumulation and vacuolation within tissues, especially neurons and epithelial cells.[86] Horses can acquire a taste for the plant and other pasture mates may actually learn their plant-seeking behavior. Plants are commonly found on heavily grazed pastures, and for unknown reasons toxicity varies with season and location.[87] The exact amount of ingested plant needed to cause toxicity varies according to species and individual susceptibility.[87] Any grazing horse can be affected initially with depression, hypersensitivity to handling, and mild incoordination. Continued exposure leads to increased severity of signs including continuous head nodding, rhythmic lip motion, abnormal tail position, emaciation due to dysphagia, and hyperreactivity.[88] In one outbreak, 9 of 25 affected horses were killed after a mild snowstorm caused manic behavior leading to severe self-trauma against the pasture fence.[88] Treatment is not often successful and affected horses usually show no clinical improvement despite removal from the affected pasture, unless performed at the very earliest sign of disease.[89] Somnolent-appearing horses should be handled with caution as they can become agitated without warning.[90,91] Diagnosis is typically made at necropsy with widespread vacuolation and degeneration of neurons in the brain. Serum biochemical changes, including depressed alpha-mannosidase and increased aspartate aminotransferase and alkaline phosphatase, as well as sporadic changes in lactate dehydrogenase, sodium, chloride, magnesium, and albumin, may be seen.[86] CSF protein was unremarkable in 3 experimentally affected yearlings.[92] Prevention involves good pasture management and lack of access for previously exposed horses that can retain the desire to eat locoweeds. Finally, lack of salt may encourage plant ingestion; therefore, access to a salt block should be provided.[91]

EQUINE NIGROPALLIDAL ENCEPHALOMALACIA (ENE)—CENTAUREA SOLSTITIALIS (YELLOW STAR THISTLE) OR ACROPTILON REPENS (RUSSIAN KNAPWEED)

Both Yellow Star Thistle (YST) and Russian Knapweed (RK) are found primarily in the western United States, frequently in dry pastures. Intoxications can occur even after drying, but horses must consume large quantities to show signs. Signs can occur after 28 days of exposure due to loss of dopaminergic neurons of the substantia nigra and globus pallidus.[92] The exact toxic principle in YST is debated and recent work focuses on 2 different theories. The first is that the presence of 2 excess neuroexcitotoxic compounds, aspartic and glutamic acids, in YST lead to death of the dopaminergic neurons.[93] However, recent work could not confirm excess excitotoxic

Table 1
Less common toxins, toxic plants, and adverse drug reactions affecting the equine nervous system

Compound	Clinical Signs	Further Reading
Alpha$_2$-adrenoreceptor agonists (xylazine, detomidine)	Unprovoked aggressive behavior	Peters DF, Erfle JB, Slobojan GT. Aggressive behavior associated with the use of xylazine and detomidine. Paper presented at 44th Annual Convention of the American Association of Equine Practitioners, 1998.
Aminophylline and theophylline	Tactile, visual, auditory hypersensitivity, muscle tremors, sweating	Errecalde JO, Button C, Mülders MS. Some dynamic and toxic effects of theophylline in horses. J Vet Pharmacol Ther 1985;8:320–7.
Blister beetle (cantharidin)	Tremors, aggression, violent, seizure-like muscular activity, head-pressing, depression, disorientation	Helman RG, Edwards WC. Clinical features of blister beetle poisoning in equids: 70 cases (1983–1996). J Am Vet Med Assoc 1997;211:1018–21.
Blue-green algae (Aphanizomenon, Anabaena, flos-aquae)	Tremors, ataxia, mydriasis, salivation, acute death, respiratory distress	Smith MO, George LW. Diseases producing cortical signs. In: Smith BP, editor. Large animal internal medicine 4th edition. St. Louis, MO: Mosby, 2009. p. 1038–9.
Bracken fern (Pteridium aquilirum), horsetail (Equisetum hypemale, Equisetum arvense)	Ataxia, weight loss, abnormal sweating, crouching stance with head and neck arched	Galey FD. Plants and other natural toxicants. In: Smith BP, editor. Large animal internal medicine, 4th edition. St. Louis, MO: Mosby, 2009. p. 1698–9.
Buckeye (Aesculus sp)	Incoordination, twitching, depression, paralysis, coma, death	Williams MC, Olsen JD. Toxicity of seeds of three Aesculus spp to chicks and hamsters. Am J Vet Res 1984;45:539–42.
Canary grass (Phalaris sp)	Collapse, convulsions, sudden heart failure, severe agitation, sudden death	Colegate SM, Anderton N, Edgar J, et al. Suspected blue canary grass (Phalaris coerulescens) poisoning of horses. Aust Vet J. 1999;77:537–8. Bourke CA, Colegate SM, Slattery S, et al. Suspected Phalaris paradoxa (paradoxa grass) poisoning in horses. Aust Vet J 2003;81:635–7.
Death Camus (Zigadenus sp)	Ataxia, stiffness, trembling, uncontrolled running, recumbency, opisthotonus, convulsions, salivation	Galey FD. Plants and other natural toxicants. In: Smith BP, editor. Large animal internal medicine, 4th edition. St. Louis, MO: Mosby, 2009. p. 1696. Cheeke PR. Natural toxicants in feeds, forages, and poisonous plants. 2nd edition. Danville, IL: Interstate Publishers; 1998. p. 393.

(continued on next page)

Table 1
(continued)

Compound	Clinical Signs	Further Reading
Dutchman's breeches (*Dicentra*)	Trembling, uncontrolled running with abnormally high head position, salivation, convulsions, recumbency, opisthotonus	
Ear tick (*Otobius megnini*)	Severe muscle cramping, percussion contracture, third eyelid prolapse	Madigan JE, Valberg SJ, Ragle C, et al. Muscle spasms associated with ear tick (Otobius megnini) infestations in five horses. J Am Vet Med Assoc 1995;207:74-6.
Fluoroquinolones (ie, enrofloxacin)	Disorientation, seizures, ataxia	Petri WA. Sulfonamides, trimethoprim-sulfamethoxazole, quinolones, and agents for urinary tract infections. In: Hardman JG, Limbird LE, Gilman AG, editors. The pharmacological basis of therapeutics, 10th edition. New York, NY: McGraw-Hill, 2001. p. 1179–84.
Jamaican nettletree (*Trema micrantha*)	Depression, locomotor deficits, blindness, recumbency, paddling, coma, and death	Bandarra PM, Pavarini SP, Raymundo DL, et al. Trema micrantha toxicity in horses in Brazil. Equine Vet J 2010;42(5):456–9.
Larkspur (*Delphinium*)	Nervousness, ataxia, salivation, arrhythmia, respiratory distress, paralysis, convulsions, and death	Galey FD. Plants and other natural toxicants. In: Smith BP, editor. Large animal internal medicine, 4th edition. St. Louis, MO: Mosby, 2009. p. 1695.
Lead	Incoordination, tremors, dysphagia, labial and anal sphincter paresis, pharyngeal paresis, CNS depression, anorexia, weight loss, anemia	Burrows GE, Borchard RE. Experimental lead toxicosis in ponies: comparison of the effects of smelter effluent-contaminated hay and lead acetate. Am J Vet Res 1982;43:2129–33.
Lidocaine	Muscle tremors, ataxia, seizure, somnolence	Meyer GA, Lin HC, Hansen RR, et al. Effects of intravenous lidocaine overdose on cardiac electrical activity and blood pressure in the horse. Equine Vet J 2001;33:434–7.

(continued on next page)

Table 1
(continued)

Compound	Clinical Signs	Further Reading
Marijuana (*Cannabis sativa*)	Depression, ataxia, agitation, vocalization, diarrhea, hypersalivation, mydriasis, urinary incontinence, seizures, and coma	
Metronidazole	Tremors, ataxia, disorientation, peripheral sensory neuronopathy, nystagmus, seizures	Dow SW, LeCouteur RA, Poss ML, et al. Central nervous system toxicosis associated with metronidazole treatment of dogs: five cases (1984–1987). J Am Vet Med Assoc 1995;195:365–8.
Milkweed (*Asclepias* sp)	Mydriasis, weakness, tremors, ataxia, convulsions, death	Burrows GE, Tyrl RJ. Plants causing sudden death in livestock. Vet Clin North Am Food Anim Pract (Clin Toxicol) 1989;5:263.
Monkshood (*Aconitum*)	Paresthesia, weakness, loss of sensation, death	Chan TY. Aconite poisoning. Clin Toxicol (Phila) 2009;47:279–85.
Mycotoxins and their respective plant source: *Rhizoctonia leguminicola* (legumes); *Acremonium lolii* (perennial ryegrass), *Claviceps paspali* (Dalis grass)	Tremors, convulsions, recumbency, depression, ataxia, death	Plumlee KH, Galey FD. Neurotoxic mycotoxins: a review of fungal toxins that cause neurological disease in large animals. J Vet Intern Med 1994;8(1):49–54. Grewar JD, Allen IG, Guthrie AJ. Annual ryegrass toxicity in Thoroughbred horses in Ceres in the Western Cape Province, South Africa. J S Afr Vet Assoc 2009;80:220–3.
Nightshades (*Atropa* sp, *Solanum* sp)	Obtundation, progressive muscular weakness, tremors, respiratory distress, tachycardia, weak pulse, ataxia, paralysis of the rear legs, coma, renal failure, death	Greer, FG. Poisoning in the horse by Woody Nightshade (Solanum dulcamara). Vet Rec 1947;45:626.
Organophosphates	Laryngeal paralysis, diarrhea, miosis, salivation, bronchoconstriction, tremors, behavioral change, seizures, generalized muscle weakness, delayed ataxia of the pelvic limbs	Duncan ID, Brook D. Bilateral laryngeal paralysis in the horse. Equine Vet J 1985;17:228–33.

(continued on next page)

Table 1
(continued)

Compound	Clinical Signs	Further Reading
Poison hemlock (*Conium maculatum*)	Muscular weakness, ataxia, tremors, central nervous system stimulation, death	Panter KE, Keeler RF, Baker DC. Toxicoses in livestock from the hemlocks (Conium and Cicuta spp.). J Anim Sci 1988;66:2407–13.
Quinidine	Nasal edema, wheals, laminitis, colic, ataxia, apprehension, mild depression	Muir WW 3rd, Reed SM, McQuirk SM. Treatment of atrial fibrillation in horses by intravenous administration of quinidine. J Am Vet Med Assoc 1990;197:1607–10. Reef VB, McGuirk SM. Disease of the cardiovascular system. In: Smith BP, editor. Large animal internal medicine, 4th edition. St. Louis, MO: Mosby, 2009. p. 485.
Rayless goldenrod (*Haplopappus heterophyllus*)	Obtundation, arched back, stiff-legged gait, tremors, weakness, collapse	Nicholson SS. Tremorgenic syndromes in livestock. Vet Clin North Am Food Anim Pract 1989;5:291–300.
Selenium	Dyspnea, diarrhea, ataxia, recumbency, blindness, circling, death	T-dargatz JL, Hamar DW. Selenium toxicity in horses. Compend Cont Educ 1986;8:771.
Stinging nettle (*Urtica dioica*)	Ataxia, muscle weakness, marked urticaria, agitation	Bathe AP. An unusual manifestation of nettle rash in three horses. Vet Rec 1994;134:11–2.
Strychnine	Rigidity, inducible tetanic seizures, recumbency, sweating, ataxia	Plumlee KH. Toxicology of organic compounds. In: Smith BP, editor. Large animal internal medicine, 4th edition. St. Louis, MO: Mosby, 2009. p. 1715.
Sudan grass (*Sorghum bicolor*)	Severe ataxia, dysuria, pollakiuria, urinary incontinence, signs of cauda equina syndrome, abortion	Morgan SE, Johnson B, Brewer B, et al. Sorghum cystitis ataxia syndrome in horses. Vet Hum Toxicol 1990;32:582. Adams LG, Dollahite JW, Romane WM, et al. Cystitis and ataxia associated with sorghum ingestion by horses. J Am Vet Med Assoc 1969;155:518–24.

(continued on next page)

Table 1
(continued)

Compound	Clinical Signs	Further Reading
Sulfer-containing plants (rape, turnip [*Brassica rapus*], fireweed [*Kochia scoparia*])	Signs of polioencephalomalacia	Douglas WW. Histamine and 5-hydroxytryptamine (serotonin) and their antagonists. In: Gilman AG, Goodman LS, Rall TW, Murad F, editors. The pharmacological basis of therapeutics, 10th edition. New York, NY: MacMillan, 1985. p. 1702.
Tobacco (*Nicotiana sp*)	Agitation, ataxia, paralysis, clonic and tonic convulsions, tremors, weak pulse, diaphragmatic paralysis	Sanecki R, Gupta RC, Kadel WL. Lethal nicotine intoxication in a group of mules. J Vet Diagn Invest 1994;6:503–4.
Water hemlock (*Cicuta maculata*)	Tremors, weakness, salivation, nervousness, convulsions, ataxia, sudden death	Panter KE, Keeler RF, Baker DC. Toxicoses in livestock from the hemlocks (Conium and Cicuta spp.). J Anim Sci 1988;66:2407–13.
White snakeroot (*Eupatorium rugosum*)	Tremors, ataxia, salivation, heavy sweating, convulsions, myopathy	Olson CT, Keller WC, Gerken DF, et al. Suspected tremetol poisoning in horses. J Am Vet Med Assoc 1984;85:1001–3.

amino acids in YST.[94] The second theory involves the inhibitory effect of repin (found in YST) on the system responsible for reducing cellular oxidants produced during routine cellular functions.[95] Repin decreases glutathione levels, increasing the susceptibility of dopaminergic neurons to oxidative damage, mitochondrial dysfunction, and death.[95] Specific deficiencies involving cranial nerves V, VII, and XII are most common and manifest as hypertonicity of facial and lip muscles, with the upper lips often pulled over the teeth in a grimace. While horses are often still able to make chewing motions, they fail to move food boluses into the back of the throat for swallowing. The retained ability to withdraw the tongue and lack of flaccid paralysis help distinguish this from botulism. Other clinical signs observed are tongue lolling, yawning, tremors, ataxia, yawning, hyperexcitability, somnolence, and head tossing.[96,97] Affected horses may attempt to drink water by immersing their head, allowing water to reach the pharynx for swallowing. Prognosis is uniformly poor and humane euthanasia is warranted as horses can perish from malnourishment and dehydration without intensive supportive care. Suspicion of ENE occurs with classic signs and history of probable exposure, but definitive diagnosis was historically only made via histopathology. Labwork is nonspecific and CSF analysis can be unremarkable.[97] This made treatment recommendations difficult as owners committed considerable finances while waiting for diagnostic tests to rule out other, potentially treatable, differential diagnoses. However, a recent report demonstrated ante-mortem diagnosis of ENE with magnetic resonance imaging.[97] Ante-mortem diagnosis allows a confident recommendation of euthanasia in a timely manner. Prevention is difficult as herbicidal removal can be costly and horses can develop a taste for the plant.[98] There is evidence of a protective effect of antioxidants such as co-enzyme Q10 and L-ascorbic acid on the toxic effects of these plants[95] and horses that must graze contaminated pastures may benefit from supplementation.

SUMMARY

This article provides an overview of the more common toxins and adverse drug reactions, along with more rare toxins and reactions (**Table 1**), that result in neurologic dysfunction in horses. A wide variety of symptoms, treatments, and outcomes are seen with toxic neurologic disease in horses. An in-depth history and thorough physical examination are needed to determine if a toxin or adverse drug reaction is responsible for the clinical signs. Once a toxin or adverse drug reaction is identified, the specific antidote, if available, and supportive care should be administered promptly.

REFERENCES

1. Humeau Y, Doussau F, Grant NJ, et al. How botulinum and tetanus neurotoxins block neurotransmitter release. Biochimie 2000;82(5):427–46.
2. Wylie CE, Proudman CJ. Equine grass sickness: epidemiology, diagnosis, and global distribution. Vet Clin North Am Equine Pract 2009;25(2):381–99.
3. Hunter J, Rohrbach BW, Andrews FM, et al. Round bale grass hay: a risk factor for botulism in horses. Compend Contin Educ Pract Vet 2002;24:166–9.
4. Kinde H, Bettey RL, Ardans A, et al. Clostridium botulinum type-C intoxication associated with consumption of processed alfalfa hay cubes in horses. J Am Vet Med Assoc 1991;199(6):742–6.
5. Schoenbaum MA, Hall SM, Glock RD, et al. An outbreak of type C botulism in 12 horses and a mule. J Am Vet Med Assoc 2000;217(3):365–8, 340.

6. Johnson AL, McAdams SC, Whitlock RH. Type A botulism in horses in the United States: a review of the past ten years (1998–2008). J Vet Diagn Invest 2010;22(2): 165–73.

7. Semrad S PS. Equine botulism. Compend Contin Educ Pract Vet 2002;24:169–172.

8. Wilkins PA, Palmer JE. Mechanical ventilation in foals with botulism: 9 cases (1989–2002). J Vet Intern Med 2003;17(5):708–12.

9. Wilkins PA, Palmer JE. Botulism in foals less than 6 months of age: 30 cases (1989–2002). J Vet Intern Med 2003;17(5):702–7.

10. Lindstrom M, Korkeala H. Laboratory diagnostics of botulism. Clin Microbiol Rev 2006;19(2):298–314.

11. Szabo EA, Pemberton JM, Gibson AM, et al. Application of PCR to a clinical and environmental investigation of a case of equine botulism. J Clin Microbiol 1994;32(8): 1986–91.

12. Yu YZ, Zhang SM, Wang WB, et al. Development and preclinical evaluation of a new F(ab') antitoxin against botulinum neurotoxin serotype A. Biochimie 2010;92(10): 1315–20.

13. Midura TF. Update: infant botulism. Clin Microbiol Rev 1996;9(2):119–25.

14. Snavely SR, Hodges GR. The neurotoxicity of antibacterial agents. Ann Intern Med 1984;101(1):92–104.

15. Center for Disease Control and Prevention (CDC). Botulism in the United States, 1899–1996. Atlanta, GA: Centers for Disease Control and Prevention; 1998.

16. Frey J, Eberle S, Stahl C, et al. Alternative vaccination against equine botulism (BoNT/C). Equine Vet J 2007;39(6):516–20.

17. Stahl C, Unger L, Mazuet C, et al. Immune response of horses to vaccination with the recombinant Hc domain of botulinum neurotoxin types C and D. Vaccine 2009; 27(41):5661–6.

18. Adam-Castrillo D, White NA 2nd, Donaldson LL, et al. Effects of injection of botulinum toxin type B into the external anal sphincter on anal pressure of horses. Am J Vet Res 2004;65(1):26–30.

19. Adinoff B, Devous MD Sr, Cooper DC, et al. Neural response to lidocaine in healthy subjects. Psychiatry Res 2009;173(2):135–42.

20. Marshall AB. Penicillin: suspected adverse reaction. Vet Rec. Mar 1 1980;106(9): 207–8.

21. Nielsen IL, Jacobs KA, Huntington PJ, et al. Adverse reaction to procaine penicillin G in horses. Aust Vet J 1988;65(6):181–5.

22. Olsen L, Ingvast-Larsson C, Brostrom H, et al. Clinical signs and etiology of adverse reactions to procaine benzylpenicillin and sodium/potassium benzylpenicillin in horses. J Vet Pharmacol Ther 2007;30(3):201–7.

23. Araszkiewicz A, Rybakowski JK. Hoigne's syndrome, kindling, and panic disorder. Depress Anxiety 1996;4(3):139–43.

24. Muir WHI. Complications: induction, maintenance and recovery phases of anaesthesia. St. Louis, MO: Mosby Year Book; 1991.

25. Holbrook TC, Dechant JE, Crowson CL. Suspected air embolism associated with post-anesthetic pulmonary edema and neurologic sequelae in a horse. Vet Anaesth Analg 2007;34(3):217–22.

26. Bueno AC, Moore RM, Seahorn TL, et al. Transient weakness, ataxia, and recumbency associated with catheterization of the right side of the heart in three horses. J Equine Vet Sci 1999;19:719–22.

27. Eckenhoff RG, Parker JW. Latency in onset of decompression sickness on direct ascent from air saturation. J Appl Physiol 1984;56(4):1070–5.

28. Bradbury LA, Archer DA, Dugdale AHA, et al. Suspected venous air embolism in a horse. Vet Rec 2005;156(5):152.
29. Gabel AA, Koestner A. The effects of intracarotid artery injection of drugs in domestic animals. J Am Vet Med Assoc 1963;142:1397–403.
30. Valentine BA, Riebold TW, Wolff PL, et al. Cerebral injury from intracarotid injection in an alpaca (Vicugna pacos). J Vet Diagn Invest 2009;21(1):149–52.
31. Christian RG, Mills JH, Kramer LL. Accidental intracarotid artery injection of promazine in the horse. Can Vet J 1974;15(2):29–33.
32. Helper LC LD. Unilateral retinopathy and blindness in a horse follwoing intracarotid injection of phenylbutazone. Equine Pract 1980;2:33–5.
33. Ponzio F, Achilli G, Calderini G, et al. Depletion and recovery of neuronal monoamine storage in rats of different ages treated with reserpine. Neurobiol Aging 1984;5(2):101–4.
34. Faria RR, Abilio VC, Grassl C, et al. Beneficial effects of vitamin C and vitamin E on reserpine-induced oral dyskinesia in rats: critical role of striatal catalase activity. Neuropharmacology 2005;48(7):993–1001.
35. Lloyd KC, Harrison I, Tulleners E. Reserpine toxicosis in a horse. J Am Vet Med Assoc 1985;186(9):980–1.
36. Bidwell LA, Schott HC, Derksen FJ. Reserpine toxicosis in an aged gelding. Equine Vet Educ 2007;19(7):341–3.
37. Anderson MA, Wachs T, Henion JD. Quantitative ionspray liquid chromatographic/tandem mass spectrometric determination of reserpine in equine plasma. J Mass Spectrom 1997;32(2):152–8.
38. Earl AE. Reserpine (serpasil) in veterinary practice. J Am Vet Med Assoc 1956;129(5):227–33.
39. Baird JD, Arroyo LG, Vengust M, et al. Adverse extrapyramidal effects in four horse given fluphenazine decanoate. J Am Vet Med Assoc 2006;229(1):104–10.
40. Brashier M. Fluphenazine-induced extrapyramidal side effects in a horse. Vet Clin North Am Equine Pract 2006;22(1):e37–45.
41. Rosengarten H, Schweitzer JW, Friedhoff AJ. A mechanism underlying neuroleptic induced oral dyskinesias in rats. Pol J Pharmacol 1993;45(4):391–8.
42. Brewer BD, Hines MT, Stewart JT, et al. Fluphenazine induced Parkinson-like syndrome in a horse. Equine Vet J 1990;22(2):136–7.
43. Baldessarini RJ TF. Drugs and the treatment of psychiatric disorders. 10th edition. New York, NY: McGraw-Hill Book; 2001.
44. Plummer CE, Kallberg ME, Ollivier FJ, et al. Suspected ivermectin toxicosis in a miniature mule foal causing blindness. Vet Ophthalmol 2006;9(1):29–32.
45. Swor TM, Whittenburg JL, Chaffin MK. Ivermectin toxicosis in three adult horses. J Am Vet Med Assoc 2009;235(5):558–62.
46. Leaning HD. The efficacy and safety evaluation of ivermectin as a parenteral and oral antiparasitic agent in horses. Paper presented at 29th Annual Convention of the American Association of Equine Practitioners, 1983.
47. Mellin TN, Busch RD, Wang CC. Postsynaptic inhibition of invertebrate neuromuscular transmission by avermectin B1a. Neuropharmacology 1983;22(1):89–96.
48. Garland TBE, Reagor JC, et al. Probably interaction between solanum eleagnifolium and ivermectin in horses. Wallingford, England: CAB International; 1998.
49. Seaman JT, Eagleson JS, Carrigan MJ, et al. Avermectin B1 toxicity in a herd of Murray Grey cattle. Aust Vet J 1987;64(9):284–5.
50. Muller JM, Feige K, Kastner SB, et al. The use of sarmazenil in the treatment of a moxidectin intoxication in a foal. J Vet Intern Med 2005;19(3):348–9.

51. Crandell DE, Weinberg GL. Moxidectin toxicosis in a puppy successfully treated with intravenous lipids. J Vet Emerg Crit Care (San Antonio) 2009;19(2):181–6.

52. Peek SF, Marques FD, Morgan J, et al. Atypical acute monensin toxicosis and delayed cardiomyopathy in belgian draft horses. J Vet Intern Med 2004;18(5):761–4.

53. Aleman M, Magdesian KG, Peterson TS, et al. Salinomycin toxicosis in horses. J Am Vet Med Assoc 2007;230(12):1822–6.

54. Alonso MA, Carrasco L. Molecular basis of the permeabilization of mammalian cells by ionophores. Eur J Biochem 1982;127(3):567–9.

55. Divers TJ, Kraus MS, Jesty SA, et al. Clinical findings and serum cardiac troponin I concentrations in horses after intragastric administration of sodium monensin. J Vet Diagn Invest 2009;21(3):338–43.

56. van der Linde-Sipman JS, van den Ingh TS, van nes JJ, et al. Salinomycin-induced polyneuropathy in cats: morphologic and epidemiologic data. Vet Pathol 1999;36(2):152–6.

57. Hanson LJ, Eisenbeis HG, Givens SV. Toxic effects of lasalocid in horses. Am J Vet Res 1981;42(3):456–61.

58. Kronfeld DS. Lasalocid toxicosis is inadequately quantified for horses. Vet Hum Toxicol 2002;44(4):245–7.

59. Bezerra PS, Driemeier D, Loretti AP, et al. Monensin poisoning in Brazilian horses. Vet Hum Toxicol 1999;41(6):383–5.

60. Van Vleet JF, Amstutz HE, Weirich WE, et al. Acute monensin toxicosis in swine: effect of graded doses of monensin and protection of swine by pretreatment with selenium-vitamin E. Am J Vet Res 1983;44(8):1460–8.

61. Henninger RW, Horst J. Magnesium toxicosis in two horses. J Am Vet Med Assoc 1997;211(1):82–5.

62. Golzarian J, Scott HW Jr, Richards WO. Hypermagnesemia-induced paralytic ileus. Dig Dis Sci 1994;39(5):1138–42.

63. Van Hook J. Hypermagnesemia. Crit Care Clin 1991;7:215–23.

64. L'Hommedieu CS, Nicholas D, Armes DA, et al. Potentiation of magnesium sulfate: induced neuromuscular weakness by gentamicin, tobramycin, and amikacin. J Pediatr 1983;102(4):629–31.

65. Mofenson HC, Caraccio TR. Magnesium intoxication in a neonate from oral magnesium hydroxide laxative. J Toxicol Clin Toxicol 1991;29(2):215–22.

66. Donovan EF, Tsang RC, Steichen JJ, et al. Neonatal hypermagnesemia: effect on parathyroid hormone and calcium homeostasis. J Pediatr 1980;96(2):305–10.

67. Dorman DC, Haschek WM. Fatal propylene glycol toxicosis in a horse. J Am Vet Med Assoc 1991;198(9):1643–4.

68. McClanahan S, Hunter J, Murphy M, et al. Propylene glycol toxicosis in a mare. Vet Hum Toxicol 1998;40(5):294–6.

69. van den Wollenberg L, Pellicaan CH, Muller K. [Intoxication with propylene glycol in two horses]. Tijdschr Diergeneeskd 2000;125(17):519–23.

70. Ross PF, Nelson PE, Owens DL, et al. Fumonisin B2 in cultured Fusarium proliferatum, M-6104, causes equine leukoencephalomalacia. J Vet Diagn Invest 1994;6(2):263–5.

71. Foreman JH, Constable PD, Waggoner AL, et al. Neurologic abnormalities and cerebrospinal fluid changes in horses administered fumonisin B1 intravenously. J Vet Intern Med 2004;18(2):223–30.

72. Wang E, Norred WP, Bacon CW, et al. Inhibition of sphingolipid biosynthesis by fumonisins. Implications for diseases associated with Fusarium moniliforme. J Biol Chem. 1991;266(22):14486–90.

73. Wang E, Ross PF, Wilson TM, et al. Increases in serum sphingosine and sphinganine and decreases in complex sphingolipids in ponies given feed containing fumonisins, mycotoxins produced by Fusarium moniliforme. J Nutr 1992;122(8):1706–16.

74. Ross PF, Ledet AE, Owens DL, et al. Experimental equine leukoencephalomalacia, toxic hepatosis, and encephalopathy caused by corn naturally contaminated with fumonisins. J Vet Diagn Invest 1993;5(1):69–74.

75. Grubb TL, Foreman JH, Benson GJ, et al. Hemodynamic effects of calcium gluconate administered to conscious horses. J Vet Intern Med 1996;10(6):401–4.

76. Wilkins PA, Vaala WE, Zivotofsky D, et al. A herd outbreak of equine leukoencephalomalacia. Cornell Vet 1994;84(1):53–9.

77. Cahill JI, Goulden BE, Jolly RD. Stringhalt in horses: a distal axonopathy. Neuropathol Appl Neurobiol 1986;12(5):459–75.

78. Domange C, Casteignau A, Collignon G, et al. Longitudinal study of Australian stringhalt cases in France. J Anim Physiol Anim Nutr (Berl) 2010;94(6):712–20.

79. Araujo JA, Curcio B, Alda J, et al. Stringhalt in Brazilian horses caused by Hypochaeris radicata. Toxicon 2008;52(1):190–3.

80. Huntington PJ, Jeffcott LB, Friend SC, et al. Australian Stringhalt–epidemiological, clinical and neurological investigations. Equine Vet J 1989;21(4):266–73.

81. Armengou L, Anor S, Climent F, et al. Antemortem diagnosis of a distal axonopathy causing severe stringhalt in a horse. J Vet Intern Med 2010;24(1):220–3.

82. Slocombe RF, Huntington PJ, Friend SC, et al. Pathological aspects of Australian Stringhalt. Equine Vet J 1992;24(3):174–83.

83. Huntington PJ, Seneque S, Slocombe RF, et al. Use of phenytoin to treat horses with Australian stringhalt. Aust Vet J 1991;68(7):221–4.

84. Ralphs MH, James LF. Locoweed grazing. J Nat Toxins 1999;8(1):47–51.

85. Dorling PR, Huxtable CR, Colegate SM. Inhibition of lysosomal alpha-mannosidase by swainsonine, an indolizidine alkaloid isolated from Swainsona canescens. Biochem J 1980;191(2):649–51.

86. Stegelmeier BL, James LF, Panter KE, et al. Dose response of sheep poisoned with locoweed (Oxytropis sericea). J Vet Diagn Invest 1999;11(5):448–56.

87. Gardner DR, Molyneux RJ, Ralphs MH. Analysis of swainsonine: extraction methods, detection, and measurement in populations of locoweeds (Oxytropis spp.). J Agric Food Chem 2001;49(10):4573–80.

88. Harries WN, Baker FP, Johnston A. Case report. An outbreak of locoweed poisoning in horses in Southwestern Alberta. Can Vet J 1972;13(6):141–5.

89. Stegelmeier BL, Ralphs MH, Gardner DR, et al. Serum alpha-mannosidase activity and the clinicopathologic alterations of locoweed (Astragalus mollissimus) intoxication in range cattle. J Vet Diagn Invest 1994;6(4):473–9.

90. James LF, Van Kampen KR, Staker GR. Locoweed (Astragalus lentiginosus) poisoning in cattle and horses. J Am Vet Med Assoc 1969;155(3):525–30.

91. Oehme FW, Bamx WE, Hulbert LC. Astragalus mollismus (locoweed) toxicosis of horses in western Kansas. J Am Vet Med Assoc 1968;152:271.

92. Young S, Brown WW, Klinger B. Nigropallidal encephalomalacia in horses fed Russian knapweed–Centaurea repens L. Am J Vet Res 1970;31(8):1393–404.

93. Roy DN, Peyton DH, Spencer PS. Isolation and identification of two potent neurotoxins, aspartic acid and glutamic acid, from yellow star thistle (Centaurea solstitialis). Nat Toxins 1995;3(3):174–80.

94. Moret S, Populin T, Conte LS, et al. HPLC determination of free nitrogenous compounds of Centaurea solstitialis (Asteraceae), the cause of equine nigropallidal encephalomalacia. Toxicon 2005;46(6):651–7.

95. Tukov FF, Rimoldi JM, Matthews JC. Characterization of the role of glutathione in repin-induced mitochondrial dysfunction, oxidative stress and dopaminergic neurotoxicity in rat pheochromocytoma (PC12) cells. Neurotoxicology 2004;25(6): 989–9.

96. Gard GP, De Sarem WG, Ahrens PJ. Nigropallidal encephalomalacia in horses in New South Wales. Aust Vet J 1973;49(2):107–8.

97. Sanders SG, Tucker RL, Bagley RS, et al. Magnetic resonance imaging features of equine nigropallidal encephalomalacia. Vet Radiol Ultrasound 2001;42(4):291–6.

98. Fowler ME. Nigropallidal encephalomalacia in the horse. J Am Vet Med Assoc 1965;147(6):607–6.

Evaluation and Management of the Recumbent Adult Horse

Rachel B. Gardner, DVM

KEYWORDS

• Recumbent • Neurologic • Sling • Down horse

DIAGNOSTIC EVALUATION
Clinical Examination

Initial evaluation of a recumbent horse involves assessment of the entire situation, including the location of the horse and safety of the horse and all involved personnel. A recumbent horse often results in a stressed environment, for both the horse and client, and it is important for the veterinarian to be observant, directive and methodical during the evaluation. Obtaining a good history can provide critical information for reaching a diagnosis as to the cause of recumbency. Signalment and a history of recent health or performance problems should be obtained. Any treatments that the horse has received should also be recorded. Onset (acute vs chronic) of the recumbency, and activity prior to the onset of recumbency should be determined. Knowledge of diet and management practices may also provide clues as to the cause of recumbency. Travel and vaccination history, especially for rabies, should be determined. Until a diagnosis is reached, all recumbent horses should be treated as rabies suspects and barrier protection used.

A thorough physical examination is paramount in the initial evaluation of a recumbent horse. Safety of the examiner is a major concern during the evaluation of the downer horse and the initial examination may best be accomplished by standing near the horse's dorsum and leaning over the body to avoid injury if the horse is thrashing its legs. The initial goal of the physical examination is to determine if the patient is stable and to determine a general cause for the recumbency. General causes of recumbency may be categorized as neurologic, musculoskeletal, cardiopulmonary, abdominal discomfort, or metabolic. In addition, initial consideration as to whether the recumbency is a result of a traumatic, infectious, metabolic, or toxic disease should be considered. Determination of this early in the examination will quickly narrow the list of differential diagnoses. A baseline respiratory rate should be obtained while the horse is undisturbed and

The author has nothing to disclose.

B.W. Furlong & Associates, PO Box 16, 101 Homestead Road, Oldwick, NJ 08858, USA

E-mail address: rgardner56@gmail.com

Vet Clin Equine 27 (2011) 527–543

doi:10.1016/j.cveq.2011.08.006

0749-0739/11/$ – see front matter © 2011 Elsevier Inc. All rights reserved.

vetequine.theclinics.com

quiet, and a baseline temperature and heart rate should be obtained. An assessment of the hydration status should also be made. The physical examination should include careful auscultation of the accessible side of the horse, including cardiopulmonary auscultation and abdominal auscultation. Palpation and manipulation of the limbs for any evidence of fracture, swelling, pain, or injury should be performed cautiously. The head and neck should also be carefully palpated for evidence of pain or fracture.

A neurologic exam, thorough to the extent possible, should be performed following physical examination. The neurologic exam should be performed systematically and results recorded throughout. The initial goal of the neurologic examination is to determine if any neurologic deficits are present and, if so, to formulate a neuroanatomic diagnosis. Initially, abnormalities may be categorized as central nervous system (CNS) disorders involving the brain and/or spinal cord, peripheral nerve system (PNS), neuromuscular junction, or multifocal disorders. A neuroanatomic diagnosis should then be made as specifically as possible so that an appropriately targeted diagnostic evaluation can be performed. The general mentation of the patient may be difficult to determine due to stress of recumbency and inability to react normally, however the horse should be evaluated closely for mental appropriateness. Observing whether the horse is interested in food and water and able to eat or drink is informative in the neurologic examination. The cranial nerve and ophthalmic exams should be performed on the accessible side, and the head may be gently lifted to evaluate the eye and cranial nerves on the recumbent side. Skin sensation and the cutaneous trunci reflex should be tested, although reliability is decreased in a recumbent horse. Focal sweating caused by sympathetic denervation may be suggestive of a lower motor neuron lesion at that site, while a unilateral or bilateral band of sweating suggests a severe thoracolumbar spinal cord lesion at the most rostral level of the sweating. If the horse can assume a dog sitting position, then injury to the spinal cord caudal to T2, myopathy, or injury to the peripheral nerves of the hindlimbs should be considered. If the horse is unable to raise the head and respiratory pattern is abnormal, either a lesion in the proximal cervical spinal cord or diffuse neuromuscular disease is likely. If the horse will only lie in lateral recumbency on one side, then vestibular disease should be considered as a cause of the recumbency. The patellar reflex should be evaluated by gently striking the middle patellar ligament to test the femoral nerve and the L4-L5 spinal cord segments. Withdrawal responses should be carefully tested by pinching the coronary band with a hemostat. A normal response in the hindlimb, characterized by flexion of the stifle and all distal joints, is achieved via the sciatic nerve and L6, S1, and S2 spinal cord segments. Withdrawal of the forelimb is achieved via the nerves of the brachial plexus and the C6-T2 spinal cord segments. Reflexes are likely to be depressed in the limbs following compression from recumbency. Tail and anal tone should be assessed, although tail tone may be altered in the recumbent horse. Bladder tone and size, and the ability to express urine from the bladder may be evaluated via rectal exam. Muscle tone, including that of the eyelid and tongue, should be evaluated carefully, as weakness is a characteristic finding with botulism.

When the recumbent physical and neurologic examinations fail to elucidate a cause for the recumbency, the horse should be assisted to stand by tail support, sling, or other means. Once assisted, many recumbent horses are able to bear weight and the cause for recumbency becomes apparent. Alternatively, abnormalities such as musculoskeletal injury or ataxia become more apparent as the horse attempts to stand with assistance.

DIAGNOSTIC TESTING

Initial diagnostic testing for any recumbent horse without a primary diagnosis should begin with a minimum database, including a complete blood count (CBC), serum biochemistry panel, and urinalysis. Anemia associated with blood loss, inadequate hematopoesis, or hemolysis, as well as anemia of chronic disease, may provide critical information in the diagnosis and treatment of the recumbent patient. Alterations of the leukogram may be indicative of inflammatory or infectious processes, although it is important to distinguish whether these changes are due to the primary disease or secondary to recumbency. Evaluation of a blood smear is always recommended to evaluate for immature or toxic neutrophils, alterations in red blood cell morphology, evidence of neoplastic cells, or infection with *Anaplasma phagocytophilum*.

Alterations in the serum biochemistry panel may also provide evidence of systemic primary disease or changes secondary to recumbency. Azotemia should be classified as prerenal (dehydration), renal (renal insufficiency), or postrenal (urinary obstruction). Myoglobinuria associated with primary myopathies or secondary to recumbency may cause acute renal failure. Significantly elevated creatine phosphokinase (CK), aspartate aminotransferase (AST), and lactate dehydrogenase (LDH) concentrations will occur with rhabdomyolysis, and to varying degrees with recumbency alone. Elevations in gamma-glutamyltransferase, AST, sorbitol dehydrogenase, lactate dehydrogenase, and bilirubin may be present with hepatic disease. It is important that an elevation in total bilirubin alone not necessarily be interpreted as evidence of hepatic disease, as anorexia may cause significant elevations in bilirubin. Hyperproteinemia may occur due to dehydration or secondary to hyperglobulinemia. Hyperglobulinemia may be suggestive of chronic infection, inflammation, or neoplasia. Panhypoproteinemia or hypoalbuminemia may occur secondary to protein loss, most commonly via the gastrointestinal tract or kidney or into a third space. Glucose concentration should also be evaluated. Although hypoglycemia may accompany a variety of systemic disorders in foals that may predispose to recumbency, the stress of disease and recumbency most often results in hyperglycemia in adult horses.

Electrolyte concentrations should be evaluated for the purposes of diagnosis of the primary cause of recumbency and for guiding therapy. At a minimum, measurement of serum sodium, potassium, chloride, and calcium concentrations is recommended. Urinalysis provides information on hydration status, renal sufficiency, proteinuria, and evidence of cystitis.

Measurement of lactate concentrations is commonly used as a marker of tissue hypoxia, disease severity and tissue perfusion. Blood ammonia may be indicated to evaluate for hepatic encephalopathy or primary hyperammonemia. Samples must be evaluated immediately or within 1 hour if kept on ice, as ammonia is unstable in blood.

Testing for specific disease processes using titers, virus isolation, and polymerase chain reaction (PCR) testing is commonly indicated in the evaluation of the recumbent horse. These tests will be discussed in further detail later.

If neurologic signs arising from the CNS are observed on examination, or if a neurologic cause of recumbency cannot be ruled out based on exam findings, evaluation of cerebrospinal fluid (CSF) may be indicated. CSF is most easily and reliably obtained via atlanto-occipital (AO) puncture in the recumbent horse. This procedure, however, requires short-term general anesthesia, so it should only be performed on a stable patient. Short-term general anesthesia using xylazine, diazepam and ketamine provides 20 to 25 minutes of anesthesia time which is adequate for the procedure. If a short-acting anesthetic was used to safely remove the horse from the transporting van/trailer, then movement of the horse and CSF collection, if desirable, can performed with a single anesthetic episode. In patients that are not considered stable for anesthesia or general anesthesia is not desired, lumbosacral puncture may be performed. The procedure is more challenging in the recumbent horse, but may be assisted via the use of ultrasound to evaluate the lumbosacral space.[1] Placing an object between the hind feet so that the legs are positioned a normal distance apart may help ensure a successful centesis. Cytologic evaluation should be provided on fresh samples. Samples may also be cultured or tested for specific antibodies/organisms if indicated.

Other diagnostic tests, such as muscle biopsy, may be useful for the diagnosis and prognosis of a recumbent patient, and will be discussed in more detail later.

Radiography using hand-held machines is useful to locate the present and extent of fractures in the limbs, head, and neck. More powerful machines may be used to locate fractures in the caudal neck, ribs, thoracolumbar vertebrae, or pelvis. Computed tomography (CT) or magnetic resonance imaging (MRI) have become more accessible to the veterinarian for evaluating the presence and severity of soft tissue and bone changes. CT and MRI remain relatively expensive and require general anesthesia, and evaluation remains limited to the head, cranial neck, and distal limbs in most average-sized equines with currently available equipment.

Ultrasonography is used in the recumbent patient to evaluate soft tissue structures, superficial bone integrity, and for the presence of body cavity effusions or hemorrhage. Endoscopy is used for evaluation of the upper airway, guttural pouches, and stylohyoid bones. An electrocardiogram is indicated in patients whose recumbency may be related to arrhythmias, or in patients in whom an arrhythmia is ausculted.

Myelography is indicated to evaluate for cervical spinal cord compression. Ventral-dorsal views are difficult to obtain in full-sized horses without a table and Bucky tray, so focal lateral sites of compression can be inapparent on routine myelography. General anesthesia and myelography should be avoided in patients that are unstable or in patients for whom a vertebral fracture remains a differential diagnosis.

Transcranial magnetic stimulation is used to measure abnormal nerve conduction along the descending motor tracts to determine the presence of a spinal cord or peripheral nerve injury.[2] Electromyography and nerve conduction velocity testing may help classify neuropathies, myopathies, or neuromuscular disorders. Electroencephalography can be used to compliment the clinical exam in identifying functional disturbances in brain activity.[3]

DIFFERENTIAL DIAGNOSES FOR RECUMBENCY

There are a myriad of diseases or disorders that may result in recumbency, and diagnosis is critical in forming a therapeutic plan and reasonable prognosis. Recumbency is a stressful situation for the horse and is frequently expensive for the client; therefore, achievement of a diagnosis and prognosis should be made as quickly as possible, but a poor prognosis should not be assumed based on recumbency alone. For the purposes of this discussion, the diseases and disorders that result in recumbency are divided into the broad categories of musculoskeletal, central nervous system, peripheral nervous system, and neuromuscular, metabolic, and cardiopulmonary causes. During evaluation, it is important to remember that secondary injuries due to recumbency or struggling may be present and can complicate diagnosis of the primary disorder.

Musculoskeletal System

Musculoskeletal disorders are one of the most common causes of recumbency. Trauma, secondary to an external blow or fall, may result in long bone, pelvic, or axial skeletal fractures. Long bone fractures are commonly diagnosed via palpation and radiography, while fractures of the pelvis are diagnosed via rectal examination and/or radiography and/or ultrasonography. Fractures of the vertebral column or ribs may be suspected based on palpation and confirmed via radiography or ultrasonography, although detection of thoracolumbar fractures in large horses is difficult due to inadequate x-ray penetration. Depending on the site of the injury, fracture stabilization may be adequate to assist the horse to rise. The prognosis is variable and depends on the site and severity of the fracture.

Laminitis commonly results in excessive recumbency; however, in severe cases, it may result in complete recumbency. Severe laminitis is diagnosed via clinical and radiographic exam, as well as history of predisposing factors such as metabolic disease, toxemia, or extreme concussion/weight bearing. Abaxial nerve blocks can help to facilitate standing and further diagnostic evaluation, such as radiography and digital venography. The prognosis for severe laminitis is multifactorial, but generally poor once severe enough to result in complete recumbency.

Generalized weakness due to age, chronic disease, severe degenerative joint disease, or cachexia commonly results in recumbency. A diagnosis is usually reached based on history and physical examination findings. History and physical examination findings, including joint palpation and radiographic findings, are typically diagnostic. Treatment with anti-inflammatory drugs and analgesics, and in the case of hindlimb degenerative joint disease, epidural administration of medications, may be sufficient to assist a patient to stand. Although many of these horses can be functional once assisted to stand, some continue to require repeat assistance unless the underlying problem is addressed with analgesics or appropriate nutrition.

Myopathies are also relatively common causes for recumbency in the horse. Depending on the type of myopathy and the severity and muscle groups involved, myopathies may result in generalized muscle sensitivity, muscle firmness on palpation, muscle trembling, and recumbency. Muscle enzymes (creatine kinase [CK], AST, lactate dehydrogenase [LDH]) are severely elevated in horses recumbent due to a myopathy and should be differentiated from mild to moderate elevations caused by recumbency alone. In cases in which severe muscle damage is present, pigmenturia may be observed. A general treatment protocol consists of intravenous fluids to correct dehydration and provide diuresis as prophylaxis against pigment nephropathy. Hypochloremia and alkalosis are common; therefore, 0.9% NaCl with supplemental potassium is recommended. Other treatments include analgesics (phenylbutazone or flunixin meglumine), intravenous DMSO, acepromazine, and methocarbamol. All of these treatments may be necessary for horses with severe exertional myopathy that become recumbent. Recumbency due to exertional myopathy may be common in exhausted horses or horses that are cast for prolonged periods. These are often the most severe myopathies seen. Horses with polysaccharide storage myopathy may also become recumbent following a severe episode. Diagnosis is based on signalment, history, elevated CK and AST concentrations, and muscle biopsy of the semimembranosus or semitendinosus muscle revealing excessive and abnormal polysaccharide accumulation with periodic acid–Schiff stain. Diagnosis of horses with the genetic (type 1) form of PSSM can be made by testing for a mutation in the gene encoding glycogen synthase 1. Quarter Horse and draft breeds are most commonly affected with type 1 PSSM. Testing is available through the Veterinary Diagnostics

Laboratory at the University of Minnesota. In addition to analgesics, recumbent PSSM horses should be treated with corn oil (6 oz/450 kg) via nasogastric tube. There are anecdotal reports of recumbent PSSM horses responding to intra-lipid infusions. If the horse becomes recumbent following anesthesia and malignant hyperthermia is a concern, treatment should also include dantrolene or phenytoin. When able to stand, management includes a low starch, high fat diet, and long-term management with regular exercise. Selenium deficiency may also result in myopathy and severe rhabdomyolysis. Involvement of the masseter and/or pterygoid muscle groups may also be observed. Further diagnostic testing includes measurement of whole blood selenium concentrations or glutathione peroxidase activity. If white muscle disease is suspected, an intramuscular injection of vitamin E/selenium should be given. Even if the presumptive diagnosis is incorrect and selenium concentration is found to be normal, a single injection of selenium given intramuscularly is unlikely to cause harm. If the diagnosis is correct, a second treatment with vitamin E/selenium 3 days later is recommended. Continued supplementation with oral selenium should be recommended. Immune mediated myositis can occur following infection with *Streptococcus equi* or viral infection. Diagnosis is by historical findings and consistent histopathologic changes in muscle biopsies. Additional treatments include corticosteroids (pred-nisolone or dexamethasone) and penicillin if *S equi* is suspected. If the immune mediated myopathy is severe and rapidly progressive, large doses (0.2 mg/kg) of dexamethasone may be required. Anaplasma myopathy is best treated with tetracycline intravenously.

Clostridial myonecrosis may occur following traumatic wounds, surgery, parturi-tion, and injections or occasionally following tissue trauma without skin penetration. Germination of clostridial spores and subsequent toxin production leads to severe tissue necrosis and possible recumbency. Fluid accumulation and gas crepitation may be palpable in the area of infection. Initial diagnosis is made based on clinical signs and history and confirmed based on anaerobic culture of the organism from the site. An ultrasound examination of the affected muscles may reveal hypoechoic areas of edema and necrosis as well as hyperechoic areas that are consistent with gas accumulation within muscles. Additional treatment consists of medications to ad-dress endotoxemia, properly dosed penicillin, metronidazole, and surgical debride-ment or fenestration to oxygenate the anaerobic environment. The prognosis is poor in severe cases with large areas of affected muscle; however, survival is possible with early and aggressive therapy.

Atypical myopathy, a peracute myopathy resulting in recumbency, has been observed most commonly in Europe but is believed to also be present in the United States.[4] The disease is more common in cooler climates and a toxin produced by either *Clostridium sordelii* or the maple leaf tar spot is suspected as a cause. Cases typically occur in the fall and spring, especially when wet weather predominates. Diagnosis is by history, clinical signs, and histologic evidence of muscle degeneration and necrosis. Treatment is supportive, although prognosis is poor once recumbency occurs.

Horses are extremely sensitive to the toxic effects of monensin, which result in skeletal and cardiac myopathy due to mitochondrial dysfunction following sodium, potassium, and calcium fluxes across the sarcolemmal membrane of muscle cells.[5] Clinical findings include ataxia, colic, weakness, tachyarrhythmias, heart failure, recumbency, and acute death. The prognosis for survival is poor in horses that have become recumbent, although horses that survive may return to athletic function.[6] Salinomycin toxicity may produce recumbency without cardiac failure.

Ingestion of white snakeroot is a possible cause of recumbency in the horse. The toxic principals of white snake root are believed to be tremetol and several other structurally related compounds. These result in alteration of the tricarboxylic acid cycle and decreased use of glucose leading to severe myonecrosis.[7] Clinical signs include weakness depression, trembling, sweating, salivation, arrhythmias, heart failure, and recumbency. The prognosis for survival once recumbency occurs is poor.

Central Nervous System

Central nervous system (CNS) disorders are also a common cause for recumbency in the horse. Supportive care for recumbent horses with CNS disorders includes judicious use of intravenous fluids, anti-inflammatory treatment with corticosteroids or NSAIDs, mannitol, intravenous DMSO, and vitamin E supplementation for antioxidant purposes.

CNS trauma may involve the brain, brainstem, or spinal cord. Abnormal findings on the neurologic exam may be a result of direct injury to the tissues or due to secondary injury from hemorrhage or edema formation and are variable based on the location of the injury. Young horses are especially susceptible to CNS trauma following basisphenoid fracture from rearing and flipping over. A head tilt, balance loss, blindness, recumbency, epistaxis, and hemorrhage from the ear may be seen. Adult horses are prone to vertebral fracture and spinal cord injury following a fall or external trauma. Radiography may be helpful if skull or vertebral fractures are present, and the presence of displaced fractures into the CNS warrants a poor prognosis. CT or MRI is helpful for providing a more definitive diagnosis and prognosis; however, a horse should only be placed under general anesthesia once vertebral fracture has been ruled out or stabilized. Supportive treatments to alleviate edema formation, antibiotic therapy if open fracture is present, and good nursing care are indicated. Further treatment, such as surgical intervention, is dependent upon the individual injury. If neurologic signs are secondary to edema/hemorrhage rather than direct CNS damage, a favorable prognosis for survival may be warranted as long as edema can be controlled before brain herniation occurs.

Compressive myelopathy may result in recumbency when involving the cervical or thoracolumbar spinal cord. Recumbency due to cervical compressive myelopathy is most commonly from cervical stenosis exacerbated by acute trauma or severe flexion of the neck such as following a myelogram. Cervical stenosis occurs in young, rapidly growing horses or older horses with osteoarthosis of the cervical facets. The history may include clumsiness or tripping, as trauma frequently exacerbates preexisting compression to result in acute recumbency. If attempts are made to stand, symmetric ataxia may be apparent. Intravertebral and intervertebral sagittal diameter ratios should be calculated on survey radiographs and may suggest vertebral canal stenosis. Osteoarthritis of the articular processes, most commonly C5-6 and C6-7 in older horses, is suggestive of the disease but not necessarily diagnostic for spinal cord compression, as many older horses have arthritic changes evident on radiographs. Cerebrospinal fluid analysis is typically normal. Definitive diagnosis is by observation of impingement of the dorsal contrast column on myelography. Transcranial magnetic stimulation may also be helpful in localizing the location of the lesion. Compression can also occur from other causes, including neoplasia, hematoma, abscess, granuloma, and cyst. Cerebrospinal fluid analysis will vary and diagnosis is based on myelographic findings of an intradural or extradural mass resulting in spinal cord compression. Treatment for compressive myelopathy depends on the cause of the compression and commonly includes high doses of dexamethasone in case of acute onset or exacerbation of signs. Surgical arthrodesis is of benefit in cases of cervical stenosis or osteoarthrosis, and surgical decompression may be indicated if a soft tissue compressive mass is present. Prognosis is guarded for survival if significant improvement does not occur quickly with medical treatment.

Although early signs may be variable, infection with the viral encephalitides can cause recumbency due to encephalomyelitis. Eastern equine encephalitis (EEE), Western equine encephalitis (WEE), and Venezuelan equine encephalitis (VEE) are clinically indistinguishable and clinical signs vary from lethargy and ataxia in the early stages to recumbency and somnolence in later stages. Fever is typically present. CSF analysis reveals mononuclear to mononuclear and neutrophilic (EEE) pleocytosis, elevated protein, and xanthochromia. Antemorten diagnosis is by demonstrating increased serum titers over a 2- to 3-week period or measuring IgM antibodies. Treatments for EEE, WEE, and VEE are supportive, although dexamethasone may be used for early and/or progressive cases. Once recumbency has occurred, the prognosis for survival is poor. Vaccines are commercially available for the viral encephalitides and are effective for prevention or decreasing disease severity.

Horses affected with WNV more commonly develop spinal cord ataxia than cerebral signs and may be recumbent. Hyperesthesia and hyperexcitability may be observed, and fasciculations of the facial and head muscles are present in approximately 50% of cases. CSF analysis may be normal or may reveal xanthochromia, lymphocytic pleocytosis, and/or increased protein. Diagnosis is made by serologic testing with immunoglobulin M capture ELISA, although horses may be negative early in the course of disease. Treatment is supportive, although administration of hyper-immune plasma early in the course of infection is likely to be helpful. Prognosis is guarded once recumbency occurs, but complete recovery is possible. Commercially available vaccines are effective for prevention or decrease in disease severity and have contributed to the decline in cases seen in recent years.

Although rabies infection occurs following the bite of an infected animal, external evidence of a bite is frequently not apparent. Clinical signs are extremely variable, from ataxia and paresis to aggressiveness and recumbency. Once clinical signs are apparent, the course of the disease tends to be rapid despite a variable and sometimes prolonged incubation period. CSF may be normal or reveal a mild lymphocytic pleocytosis and/or mildly elevated protein level. No test exists for the antemortem diagnosis of rabies. No treatment is available, the disease is invariably fatal, and zoonotic potential should be considered high, so treatment of an animal in which rabies is suspected is not recommended. Any horse in which rabies remains a differential diagnosis should be treated with strict biosecurity measures. Human exposure should be limited and a list should be kept of all individuals who have had contact with the horse. Gloves should be worn and all specimens from the patient labeled with "Rabies Suspect." Commercial vaccines are available and effective for prevention.

Equine herpesvirus-1 (EHV-1) causes respiratory disease, abortion, and neurologic disease. Neurologic signs are due to CNS vasculitis and commonly cause recumbency. EHV-1 typically affects older adult horses in situations of high stocking density or increased movement of horses. Although isolated cases are occasionally seen, outbreaks are common unless quarantine measures are already in place. Affected horses are usually febrile and other horses without neurologic signs on the same farm may be febrile. Clinical findings consist of a rapid onset of symmetric ataxia that may progress to recumbency. Hindlimb ataxia is typically worse than in the forelimbs and may result in "dog sitting." Urinary bladder paralysis and urine dribbling are common. Fecal retention may occur and is more common in recumbent patients. CSF is commonly xanthochromic with an elevated protein level. Diagnosis is by history and clinical signs and is confirmed by PCR testing on whole blood and nasal swab samples. Virus isolation from nasal swabs or CSF may be performed early in the course of disease or to confirm a positive PCR result. Rising serum neutralization titers are also diagnostic, although many horses will have high titers at the onset of clinical signs. Treatment is largely supportive, although several adjunct treatments have been recommended. Moderate- to high-dose dexamethasone is recommended in rapidly progressive or severe cases. Bethanecol may be used to manage bladder distention and antibiotics are typically necessary to treat cystitis secondary to frequent urinary bladder catheterization. Valacyclovir is frequently used early in infection but beneficial effects were not demonstrated in one study.[8] The prognosis is variable, although individuals who become rapidly recumbent tend to have a poor prognosis. Strict quarantine measures should be taken when EHV-1 infection is suspected. All horses at risk should have temperatures monitored at least twice daily and febrile horses should be isolated. Febrile cases should be confirmed using PCR testing of whole blood and nasal swabs and facilities should be quarantined until at least 30 days after the last case is confirmed. Vaccination during an outbreak is not usually recommended, although vaccinating after clinical signs have resolved is suggested. The findings of fever and rapidly progressive ataxia and paresis leading to recumbency with discolored CSF could easily be confused with anaplasmosis is some areas of the country. Multiple horses developing recumbency without fever may occur with botulism, moldy corn poisoning, atypical myopathy, and ionophore toxicity.

Equine protozoal myelitis (EPM) is most commonly due to CNS infection with *Sarcocystis neurona*, although infection with other protozoal species has been reported.[9] Affected horses are most commonly between the ages of 1.5 and 4 years of age and remain afebrile. A history of stress, such as shipping or showing, is common prior to the onset of signs. Recumbency is most commonly associated with peracute or acute onset of signs and is occasionally accompanied by vestibular signs, cranial nerve signs, or signs of lower motor neuron disease of the limbs. Ataxia prior to recumbency is commonly asymmetric. CSF analysis is typically normal. Serum to CSF SAG2/3/4 ELISA titer ratios or indirect fluorescent antibody testing on serum and/or CSF is currently recommended for diagnosis.[10,11] False-negative results may occur in acute cases and retesting may be indicated. Treatment consists of supportive care and antiprotozoal medication such as ponazuril, diclazuril or a sulfadiazine-trimethoprim-pyrimethamine combination. Double doses of ponazuril are commonly used for the first week of treatment. In suspect acute cases, treatment is recommended while awaiting laboratory confirmation. Prognosis is poor once recumbency has occurred but improves with early and aggressive treatment. Relapse is possible following cessation of treatment. Although steroid therapy is controversial, both corticosteroids and DMSO may be useful in rapidly progressive cases.

Severe vestibular dysfunction may result in recumbency due to balance loss. Temporohyoid osteoarthropathy is the most common cause of severe vestibular signs in the horse and affected horses may have a history of unusual chewing behavior or an incident causing sudden head elevation. Horses with acute onset of severe peripheral vestibular signs demonstrate nystagmus (fast phase away from the lesion) and a head tilt, and prefer to lie on the side of the lesion. If the horse can be assisted to stand, circling and leaning toward the side of the lesion are observed. Strength is maintained and contralateral hypertonia may be present. Mentation remains normal and facial nerve paralysis commonly occurs simultaneously with vestibular signs. If the inflammatory process extends into the meninges, depression, weakness, and proprioceptive deficits may also be observed. Endoscopy of the guttural pouches or dorsoventral skull radiographs reveal enlargement of the proximal stylohyoid bone on the affected side. Diagnosis can be further confirmed by using CT or MRI. Treatment consists of supportive care and anti-inflammatory therapy. Otitis media and interna can cause similar signs or may occur concurrently with stylohyoid osteoarthropathy; therefore, antibiotic treatment with trimethroprim-sulfa, enrofloxacin, or chloramphenicol is recommended. If facial nerve paralysis is present, frequent ophthalmic lubrication or tarsorrhaphy is recommended. Surgical resection of the ceratohyoid bone is recommended to decrease risk of recurrence and may hasten recovery. Prognosis for temporohyoid arthropathy is fair to good in cases of strictly peripheral involvement.

Equine motor neuron disease (EMND) is an acquired neurodegenerative disorder of adult horses affecting motor neurons in the spinal cord ventral horn and brainstem. Neuronal damage results in denervation muscle atrophy, especially of type 1 (postural) muscle fibers. In the subacute stages, horses may show signs of weakness, trembling, base-narrow stance, weight loss, sweating, and excessive recumbency. Ophthalmic evaluation reveals fundic lesions from lipofuscin accumulation in approximately 30% of cases. Diagnosis is made on the basis of history and clinical findings, as well as the observation of denervation muscle atrophy in a biopsy of the sacrocaudalis dorsalis (tailhead) muscle. Chronic or historical vitamin E deficiency is thought to be the most important factor in the development of EMND, although serum vitamin E levels may be normal at the time of diagnosis. Affected horses should be administered 5000 to 7000 IU vitamin E daily, although the prognosis is poor for the uncommon recumbent horses.

Equine anaplasmosis, caused by infection with *Anaplasma phagocytophilum*, occasionally causes ataxia, which can progress to recumbency.[12] Horses are febrile and may exhibit depression, anorexia, edema, icterus, petechiae, and orchitis. Diagnosis made by observation of inclusions in neutrophils, PCR testing of whole blood, or rising serum titers. Treatment consists of tetracycline and supportive care. Response to treatment tends to be rapid and the prognosis is good.

Tetanus occurs following infection of a wound with *Clostridium tetani* and production of exotoxin that prevents the release of inhibitory neurotransmitters. It results in skeletal muscle spasticity, which causes stiffness, trembling, spasm, and recumbency. Masseter muscle stiffness, eyelid retraction, and flared nostrils are commonly present. Clinical signs are exacerbated by excitement that can result in recumbency, if not already present, and risk of secondary trauma. Diagnosis is based on clinical signs in an unvaccinated horse with a history of a soft tissue wound 1 to 3 weeks earlier. Treatment is with antitoxin administration, which binds residual circulating exotoxin. Intrathecal administration of antitoxin may be performed in early cases that remain ambulatory. If a wound is apparent, it should be debrided to oxygenate the anaerobic environment. Additional therapy consists of supportive care, maintaining a quiet environment, and tranquilization if necessary. Sedation with muscle relaxation should precede slinging or other procedures. Concurrent vaccination is indicated, as infection may not stimulate an adequate immune response. The prognosis for recumbent horses is grave.

Hepatic encephalopathy or primary hyperammonemia may occasionally result in recumbency. Clinical signs include acute cerebral signs, including behavior change, blindness, circling, seizures, and recumbency. Horses with hepatic encephalopathy have elevated liver enzyme activities, abnormal hepatic function tests, and icterus. Horses with primary hyperammonemia commonly have a history of gastrointestinal disease, most commonly colic and/or diarrhea, prior to the onset of neurologic signs. Definitive diagnosis is by measurement of elevated blood ammonia greater than 150 μmol/L. Concurrent metabolic acidosis and hyperglycemia are supportive findings.

Treatment includes treatment of liver disease if present, sedation with phenobarbital or small doses of xylazine as necessary, oral neomycin, intravenous fluid therapy, and oral magnesium sulfate. The prognosis for hepatic encephalopathy is poor due to severe liver disease; however, primary hyperammonemia has a more favorable prognosis.

Toxicities may also lead to CNS signs and recumbency. Ingestion of bracken fern causes signs of polioencephalomalacia such as lethargy, ataxia, blindness, and recumbency due to thiaminase activity. Treatment is intravenous or intramuscular thiamine administration. Ingestion of the mycotoxin fumonisin B1, found in corn and other grains infected with *Fusarium moniliforme*, causes cerebral signs and recumbency due to leukoencephalomalacia. Diagnosis is made by clinical signs and observation of infected feed, which may have a pink or brown discoloration. The prognosis is poor for horses that have become recumbent.

Adverse reactions to fluphenazine decanoate can result in recumbency due to CNS effects. Fluphenazine is a phenothiazine neuroleptic drug used as an antipsychotic to treat schizophrenia and bipolar disorder in humans. It is used in horses as a long-acting sedative. Clinical signs observed prior to recumbency may include agitation, sweating, hypermetria, circling, wide head excursions, violent pawing, and stupor.[13] Diagnosis is made based on clinical signs and a history of fluphenazine decanoate injection, although disclosure that the medication had been administered may be withheld due to illicit use of the drug. Diagnosis is confirmed by detection of the drug in serum. Treatment consists of supportive care and the administration of anticholinergics such as diphenhydramine hydrochloride or benztropine mesylate.

Inadvertent intracarotid injection of medications may result in signs of hyperexcitability, collapse, seizure, or coma. Signs may be violent and occur immediately following drug administration. Once the horse can be safely approached, treatment consists of sedation as needed, antiedema and anti-inflammatory medications, and supportive care. The prognosis is favorable for water-soluble drugs (acepromazine, detomidine, xylazine). The prognosis is poor for oil-based drugs (diazepam, procaine penicillin, phenylbutazone) and may result in immediate death. Intracarotid injection of flunixin meglumine tends to produce less severe, transient signs.

Peripheral Nervous and Neuromuscular Systems

Peripheral nerve disorders that cause recumbency result from mechanical injury or trauma, EPM gray matter disease, neoplasia, abscess, caudal aortic thrombosis, or iatrogenic causes. Abnormalities of major peripheral nerves result in muscle weakness (paresis or paralysis), hyporeflexia or areflexia, hypotonia or atonia, and neurogenic atrophy. With unilateral femoral paralysis, a horse may initially be able to bear weight on the contralateral hindlimb, but it will commonly fatigue, leading to recumbency. Bilateral femoral nerve paralysis results in recumbency and inability to stand. This is most commonly due to acute EPM or dystocia. Obturator nerve paralysis may occur following sudden and severe hindlimb abduction and results in persistent abduction and possible recumbency, especially on smooth or slippery surfaces. Diagnosis is based on clinical signs, history, and serum EPM testing. In horses recumbent due to caudal aortic thrombosis, the pelvic limbs are cold, associated muscles are firm on palpation, and no femoral pulse is present. The prognosis for recumbency due to a peripheral nerve disorder, gray matter disease or thrombosis is guarded regardless of etiology, although with early and aggressive treatment of EPM, recovery may be possible.

Botulism is frequently associated with feed contamination; cases may be seen sporadically or as an outbreak. The *C botulinum* toxin binds to presynaptic receptors at the neuromuscular junction to prevent the release of acetylcholine, resulting in lower motor neuron paralysis and weakness. The onset of recumbency may be acute or slow. Trembling occurs due to weakness when horses are standing and resolves during recumbency. Dysphagia is a common presenting sign and persists once recumbent. Diagnosis is based on history and clinical signs. Diagnosis can be confirmed by the presence of botulinum toxin in feed, serum, gastrointestinal contents, or wound contents or the presence of spores in intestinal contents. Although several tests are available, a mouse bioassay is most commonly used since it is most sensitive and only small amounts of toxin are required to produce severe clinical signs in horses. Treatment consists of administration of specific or multivalent antiserum early in the course of the disease. The prognosis is poor in adult horses once recumbency has occurred, although complete recovery is possible with excellent nursing care. Prevention of the disease is by vaccination with a type B toxoid, which is only protective against type B intoxication.

Metabolic Disorders

Disorders that lead to electrolyte abnormalities (hyponatremia, hypocalcemia, hyperkalemia) or hypoglycemia may result in recumbency. Hyperkalemia is most commonly observed during episodes of hyperkalemic periodic paralysis (HYPP) in Quarter Horses or Quarter Horse crosses, or secondary to uroperitoneum or renal failure. Clinical signs include muscle stiffness, fasciculations, muscle weakness, respiratory stridor, recumbency, and death. Cardiac arrhythmias may be detected and an electrocardiogram may reveal several changes, including peaked T waves. Diagnosis is by clinical signs and serum potassium level greater than 6 mEq/L. If signs are observed in a Quarter Horse type breed, HYPP should be highly suspected and may be later confirmed via DNA testing. Treatment for HYPP is slow intravenous administration of calcium borogluconate, $NaHCO_3$, or dextrose solution. Long-term management includes dietary management and the use of potassium-wasting diuretics such as acetazolamide.

Exhaustion occurs in horses that are overworked, especially in hot, humid conditions. In horses recumbent from exhaustion, severe sweating, tachycardia, tachypnea, severe dehydration, cardiac arrhythmias, synchronous diaphragmatic flutter, and CNS signs may be observed. Hypochloremia, hyponatremia, and hypocalcemia, as well as hemoconcentration, azotemia, hyperlactatemia, and increased muscle and liver enzyme concentrations, are commonly present on a biochemistry panel. Diagnosis is based on history and clinical signs. Treatment includes decreasing body temperature, fluid resuscitation and electrolyte replacement via intravenous and/or oral routes, NSAIDs following fluid replacement, and antiendotoxic treatments. The prognosis is good if the initial response to treatments is rewarding. Delayed onset of myopathy, laminitis, hepatic insufficiency, and renal insufficiency are possible several days following the episode.

Although more commonly observed in neonates, hypoglycemia may rarely cause episodic collapse or recumbency in the adult horse. Hypoglycemia is seen with a variety of disorders in horses; however, severe hypoglycemia associated with collapse or recumbency is most commonly secondary to tumors.[14] In humans, tumors are proposed to cause hypoglycemia due to insulin production by functional insulinomas, tumor catabolism lowering blood glucose, secretion by the tumor of insulin-like factors, interference with hepatic function, and suppression of counter-regulatory hormones.[15] Clinical signs include weakness, lethargy, muscle fasciculations, ataxia, collapse, and recumbency. Diagnosis is based on clinical signs and measurement of hypoglycemia. Treatment is intravenous and/or oral glucose supplementation; however, evaluation for a primary problem resulting in hypoglycemia should be pursued.

Respiratory and Cardiovascular Systems

Recumbency may result from respiratory conditions that result in hypoxemia. Upper airway conditions are most likely to result in acute respiratory distress and recumbency and are typically characterized by an inspiratory stridor. The differential diagnoses for the cause of the upper airway obstruction are numerous, but complete evaluation should only be attempted after the patient has been stabilized. If labored breathing and an inspiratory stridor consistent with an upper airway obstruction are observed, nasotracheal intubation or tracheotomy should be performed and oxygen insufflation provided if possible. Respiratory distress without stridor is less commonly acute in onset but could still result in recumbency. Differential diagnoses include severe pneumonia, pleuropneumonia, pneumothorax, pulmonary edema, and recurrent airway obstruction. Diagnosis is based on the presence of respiratory distress and abnormalities on auscultation of the thorax. Specific auscultation findings and treatment will vary depending on the disease process causing the recumbency.

Cardiovascular collapse, especially when acute, may result in recumbency. Hemorrhage, whether internal or external, may result in cardiovascular collapse. Internal hemorrhage occurs most commonly into the abdomen, although hemorrhage into the thorax and uterus may occur as well. Initial diagnosis is based on history, mucous membrane pallor, tachypnea, tachycardia, abdominal discomfort, and low blood pressure. Further evaluation to determine the origin of hemorrhage includes ultrasound examination and abdominocentesis or thoracocentesis. Supportive treatment includes keeping the horse quiet, administration of intravenous fluids to maintain low to normal blood pressure, blood transfusion, intravenous aminocaproic acid, NSAIDs, and intranasal oxygen insufflation. Autotransfusion may be considered with hemorrhage into a cavity in the absence of sepsis; otherwise drainage should not be performed. The prognosis is good if the hemorrhage can be controlled.

Severe shock may also cause recumbency, whether due to decreased perfusion or secondary to sepsis. Diagnosis is based on history and clinical signs of dark mucous membranes with prolonged capillary refill time, poor peripheral pulses, and cool extremities. Basic treatment of severe shock begins with reestablishment of the circulatory volume with intravenous fluids (both crystalloids and colloids) and oxygen insufflation and may include pressor agents and dobutamine. Antibiotic therapy and antiendotoxic therapies such as plasma, polymixin B, DMSO, or pentoxifylline are indicated in the case of septic shock. Even with aggressive therapy, the severity of shock required to cause recumbency in an adult horse warrants a poor prognosis.

MANAGEMENT

Transport of the recumbent horse is challenging and potentially dangerous due to the size and weight of a full-sized horse and because many recumbent horses are frightened and may react violently to being moved. In a quiet or depressed horse, transport may be carried out without the use of sedation/anesthesia; however, some degree of sedation is typically necessary in order to move a horse safely. Protection for the horse, in the form of padded leg wraps and a helmet, are useful if available. Recumbent horses can be moved on a flat surface with a coordinated effort by several people simultaneously pulling/pushing the horse in the same direction. Ropes can be tied to the down limbs to allow more distance between the limbs and people for safety. More effectively, a horse can be moved using a Large Animal Rescue Glide. The glide is a large sheet of conformable plastic with handles and areas to hook ropes around the edges. The plastic slides easily over a variety of surfaces and the edges can be folded to accommodate stall and trailer doorways. An effective method for moving a recumbent horse is to place the UC Davis Large Animal Lift, discussed in the next section, on the horse and use it to pull the horse onto a Large Animal Rescue Glide. The glide can then be pulled into a trailer for transport. With the glide in place, the horse can then be easily pulled off the trailer and into a hospital stall.

Management of the recumbent horse must include treatment of the primary disease, when known or possible, and intensive supportive care. Supportive care of the recumbent horse begins with appropriate bedding to help minimize complications such as decubital ulcers and compressive myopathies and neuropathies. Bedding should be compressible, comfortable, and absorbent and should be cleaned and aerated each time the horse is turned or moved. A base layer of absorbent wood shavings with a thick covering of straw works very well. Once the horse is able to stand or if assisted with a sling, it is important that the bedding provide solid footing and not be excessively deep. If possible, sheets or blankets may be placed on top of the straw to prevent abrasions, especially under the head. The head should be slightly elevated by means of extra bedding or blankets/pillows.

When possible, the recumbent horse should be assisted to remain in sternal, rather than lateral, recumbency, by propping up with straw or shavings bales. The horse should be turned every 2 to 6 hours, even if the horse is able to remain in sternal recumbency. Turning helps to prevent decubital ulcers, compressive myopathy, and neuropathy and supports ventilation. Turning is ideally achieved by placing the horse is sternal recumbency and pushing the body over the limbs. In full-sized horses, however, this is nearly impossible and the horse must be turned by pulling the limbs over the body. With the horse in lateral recumbency, ropes should be tied to the down limbs. With one person assisting to turn the head, the ropes should be pulled by individuals standing on the opposite side of the horse as the limbs. Care should be taken to remain a good distance from the horse since struggling frequently occurs as the horse is turned, although most horses seem to get used to the procedure over time. The bedding should be cleaned and turned prior to turning the horse. Although the "down" lung will have some degree of atelectasis, this does not typically cause a problem except in horses with botulism or with weak intercostal/diaphragm muscles.

Many recumbent horses can bear some weight if assisted to stand and can spend considerable time upright with the assistance of a sling. By increasing the time a horse stands, adverse effects of prolonged recumbency are minimized and some muscle mass can be maintained. A sling can provide the examiner with the opportunity to more effectively evaluate an otherwise recumbent patient for signs of neurologic or musculoskeletal signs to better formulate a diagnosis and/or prognosis. Patient selection is important when considering the use of a sling. Horses with abnormal mentation are not candidates for slinging and horses with fractious or nervous behavior may require the use of light sedation or tranquilization. It is imperative that a sling be adjusted properly to prevent pressure sores and fit comfortably. A horse should be monitored closely when in the sling, as collapse may cause respiratory distress and death due to pressure on the thorax and/or trachea. Initially, horses should be assisted to stand for short periods of time, and the time gradually increased if tolerated. Horses with botulism should not be assisted to stand with a sling unless necessary due to complications of recumbency.

To use a sling safely in a stall environment, a cross beam and hoist capable of supporting at least 2000 to 4000 lb should be available, depending on the size of the horse, sling, and hoist. The UC Davis-Anderson sling provides the most support in the most stable and balanced manner. This sling consists of a rectangular overhead support that provides level support and additional leg supports alleviate excessive pressure on the abdomen and thorax/sternum. Disadvantages of this sling are that it is expensive and can be difficult to place, especially on a recumbent horse without sedation or anesthesia. The Liftex sling is simpler to use, containing an abdominal support as well as tail and chest supports. It is less expensive and easier to place on the recumbent patient than the Anderson Sling. The UC Davis Large Animal Lift is more affordable and more lightweight than the previous slings. It is intended to be used for lifting and moving horses, rather than providing ongoing support for a horse unable to stand unassisted, although it can be used in this manner for short periods of time. This device is relatively simple to place on a recumbent horse and can be used with a tractor or winch for lifting. In a situation when the horse needs continued support for standing, the Anderson sling may be placed over the UC Davis Large Animal Lift once the horse has been lifted to a standing position. On an especially quiet horse, the horse may be lifted using the sling and positioned in a bovine float tank. The horse must be monitored closely and there is risk of injury while in the confined tank.

The newest device available is the Enduro NEST (NASA Equine Support Technology), developed by Enduro Medical Technology. With this equipment, the horse is supported with a sling containing an abdominal support and leg supports. The sling is supported by a self-contained metal frame to provide customized support or enable lifting of the animal. A horse can be placed under and recover from general anesthesia safely while being continuously supported in a standing position. The device can be used stationary to provide variable limb support or can be mobile to assist a weak, injured, or neurologic horse to walk.

Decubital ulcers and self-trauma are difficult to prevent but can be minimized with attention to bedding and skin care. Leg wraps are recommended to protect the distal limbs from self-trauma and shoes should be wrapped to alleviate sharp edges that result in lacerations. Well-fitting head bumpers are useful to help prevent head trauma, which commonly occurs during failed attempts to get into sternal recumbency. Horses should be groomed frequently—ideally before and after each time the horse is turned. Damp areas from sweat or urine should be dried thoroughly, as wet skin is more prone to pressure sores and ulceration. Wounds should be kept clean and dry, and antibiotics or topical medications are used if necessary.

Ophthalmic lubrication with an artificial tear ointment should be performed bilaterally at least 6 to 8 times daily. The corneas should be stained at least once daily to monitor for corneal ulceration, more frequently if blepharospasm, miosis, or a change in corneal appearance is observed. Corneal ulcers should be treated aggressively and a temporary tarsorrhaphy considered to protect the cornea.

Nutritional support is an integral and challenging aspect of supportive care for the recumbent horse. Horses that are not dysphagic should be propped into sternal recumbency and offered water and typical diets of long stem forage and grain. Horses are more likely to want to eat while standing, so feed and water should be offered at nose height when assisted to stand. Horses that are dysphagic or inappetent for several days require enteral or parenteral nutritional support. Enteral feeding may be provided via nasogastric tube, and the tube can be left indwelling or passed several times daily. Enteral diets may be formulated using complete feeds or alfalfa meal, or a commercial equine enteral diet may be used. Feedings should be divided into four to six small meals per day and administered with the horse in sternal recumbency or while standing. In horses with adequate gastrointestinal function, maintenance fluids may be provided via nasogastric tube. In horses with gastrointestinal dysfunction in which enteral feeding is not possible, parenteral nutrition with dextrose, amino acids, and lipid solutions should be considered. Maintenance fluid requirements must also be met using intravenous fluids in horses with dysphagia or inadequate gastrointestinal function.

Intravenous catheter care is challenging in recumbent horses due to an unavoidably contaminated environment and frequent motion. Polyurethane over-the-wire jugular catheters are recommended, as they are less likely to cause thrombosis than over-the-needle catheters. Flushing the catheter with heparinized saline several times daily is recommended if continuous fluids are not being administered. An Elastikon neck wrap with dry gauze placed over the base of the catheter is recommended to prevent friction and gross contamination at the catheter insertion site and should be replaced daily or when soiled. The vein and the catheter insertion site should be inspected at least twice daily for evidence of skin swelling, heat, or thickening of the vein. If any abnormalities are detected, the catheter should be removed and the tip cultured. Hot-packing the catheter site and vein several times daily, followed by topical application of DMSO/furacin sweat, icthammol, or Surpass (Boehringer Ingelheim Vetmedica, St. Joseph, MO, USA), is recommended to help minimize thrombophlebitis. Antibiotic therapy is typically indicated.

Urinary catheterization is necessary in horses with neurologic disorders that cause an atonic bladder, such as EHV-1, and in horses that do not urinate appropriately. Some recumbent horses, both males and females, may choose not to urinate even with normal bladder and spinal cord function. Catheterization may be performed several times daily, or the catheter may be left indwelling. Indwelling catheterization is useful for keeping the bedding and patient dry and helping to prevent decubital ulceration. An indwelling Foley catheter should be placed under sterile conditions and urine should be collected using a closed system. Intravenous tubing and empty sterile intravenous fluid bags placed deep in the bedding below the level of the bladder can be easily and inexpensively used for urine collection. Securing the catheter and/or tubing to the skin on the ventral body wall (males) or tail (mares) using elastic tape or suture, respectively, will alleviate pressure on the catheter when the horse struggles or is turned. The urinary collection system should be monitored for obstructions and urine collection bags emptied at least several times daily. The most common complication of urinary catheterization is cystitis due to ascending bacterial infection. Cytologic and dipstick evaluation of urine is easy and inexpensive and should be performed every few days. If cystitis is suspected (neutrophils and/or bacteria present), a urine culture and colony count should be performed and antibiotic therapy instituted.

Large colon impactions are common in recumbent horses due to poor gastrointestinal motility. Easily digestible feeds should be offered and mineral oil administered via nasogastric tube as needed to maintain soft manure. Manual evacuation of the rectum is frequently necessary, especially in horses with EHV-1.

SUMMARY

Evaluation and management of recumbent horses are challenging. Familiarity with disorders that can result in recumbency will facilitate more rapid diagnosis and more appropriate formulation of a prognosis. With rapid and appropriate diagnosis, appropriate treatment can be pursued and, with good nursing care, can result in a favorable outcome.

REFERENCES

1. Aleman M, Borchers A, Kass PH, et al. Ultrasound-assisted collection of cerebrospinal fluid from the lumbosacral space in equids. J Am Vet Med Assoc 2007;230(3): 378–84.

2. Nollet H, Vanschandevijl K, Van Ham L, et al. Role of transcranial magnetic stimulation in differentiating motor nervous tract disorders from other causes of recumbency in four horses and one donkey. Vet Rec 2005;157(21):656–8.
3. Lacombe VA, Podell M, Furr M, et al. Diagnostic validity of electroencephalography in equine intracranial disorders. J Vet Intern Med 2001;15(4):385–93.
4. Finno CJ, Valberg SJ, Wunschmann A, et al. Seasonal pasture myopathy in horses in the Midwestern United States: 14 cases (1998–2005). J Am Vet Med Assoc 2006; 229(7):1134–41.
5. Matsuoka T. Evaluation of monensin toxicity in the horse. J Am Vet Med Assoc 1976;169(10):1098–100.
6. Hughes KJ, Hoffmann KL, Hodgson DR. Long-term assessment of horses and ponies post exposure to monensin sodium in commercial feed. Equine Vet J 2009;41(1):47–52.
7. Lee ST, Davis TZ, Gardner DR, et al. Tremetone and structurally related compounds in white snakeroot (Ageratina altissima): a plant associated with trembles and milk sickness. J Agric Food Chem 2010;58(15):8560–5.
8. Garre B, Gryspeerdt A, Croubels S, et al. Evaluation of orally administered valacyclovir in experimentally EHV1-infected ponies. Vet Microbiol 2009;135(3-4):214–21.
9. Finno CJ, Aleman M, Pusterla N. Equine protozoal myeloencephalitis associated with neosporosis in 3 horses. J Vet Intern Med 2007;21(6):1405–8.
10. Reed SM, Howe DK, Yeargan MR, et al. New quantitative assays for the differential diagnosis of equine protozoal myeloencephalitis (EPM). In: Proceedings of the 2010 ACVIM Forum. California; 2010. p. 339.
11. Johnson AL, Burton AJ, Sweeney RW. Utility of 2 immunological tests for antemortem diagnosis of equine protozoal myeloencephalitis (Sarcocystis neurona infection) in naturally occurring cases. J Vet Intern Med 2010;24(5):1184–9.
12. Nolen-Walston RD, K'Oench SM, Hanelt LM, et al. Acute recumbency associated with Anaplasma phagocytophilum infection in a horse. J Am Vet Med Assoc 2004; 224(12):1964–6.
13. Baird JK, Arroyo LG, Vengust M, et al. Adverse extrapyramidal effects in four horses given fluphenazine decanoate. J Am Vet Med Assoc 2006;229(1):104–10.
14. Haga HA, Ytrehus B, Rudshaug IJ, et al. Gastrointestinal stromal tumour and hypoglycemia in a Fjord pony: a case report. Acta Vet Scand 2008;50(1):9.
15. Kahn CR. The riddle of tumour hypoglycaemia revisited. Clin Endocrinol Metab 1980;9(2):335–60.

Guttural Pouch Diseases Causing Neurologic Dysfunction in the Horse

Alexandre S. Borges, DVM, MS, PhD[a],*,
Marcos J. Watanabe, DVM, MS, PhD[b]

KEYWORDS

• Guttural pouch • Dysphagia • Mycosis • Cranial nerves

Several diseases of the guttural pouches have been described in the literature, and the comprehensive evaluation of these structures is an important element of the clinical exam. Guttural pouch abnormalities form part of an important group of differential diagnoses for horses presenting dysphagia, cough, fever, nasal discharge, epistaxis, and cranial nerve abnormalities. Endoscopy of the guttural pouches provides a unique opportunity to visualize nervous structures. Moreover, this is probably the only place where we are able to observe so many nervous structures simultaneously. There is a close anatomic relationship between the guttural pouches, cranial nerves, and sympathetic structures; therefore, several guttural pouch diseases can lead to neurologic abnormalities. Guttural pouch examination also allows evaluation of the temporohyoid joint, which aids in the differential diagnosis of vestibular or facial nerve dysfunction associated with fractures. This text will address the descriptive anatomy of the guttural pouch, emphasizing the nervous structures in direct contact with it and the possible neurologic signs resulting from disease. We will also review the major literature regarding guttural pouch diseases associated with neurologic abnormalities.

GUTTURAL POUCH ANATOMY AND NERVOUS STRUCTURES HAVING DIRECT CONTACT WITH THE GUTTURAL POUCH

The guttural pouch is an auditory tube diverticulum found in the horse and other members of the order Perissodactyla; it connects the nasopharynx to the middle ear.[1]

Disclosures: Alexandre S. Borges has a grant from the Conselho Nacional de Pesquisa CNPq. The authors have nothing to disclose.
[a] Department of Veterinary Clinical Science, College of Veterinary Medicine and Animal Science, São Paulo State University, Botucatu-SP, Zip Code 18618970, Brazil
[b] Department of Veterinary Surgery and Anesthesiology, College of Veterinary Medicine and Animal Science, São Paulo State University, Botucatu-SP, Zip Code 18618970, Brazil
* Corresponding author.
E-mail address: asborges@fmvz.unesp.br

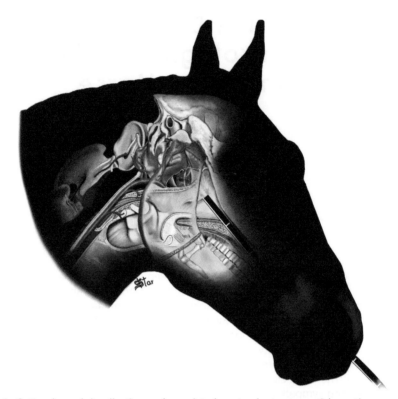

Fig. 1. Guttural pouch localization and associated anatomic structures. Schematic representation of guttural pouch extending from the base of skull and the atlas to the nasopharynx and associated anatomic structures. Left pharyngeal orifice is represented associated with endoscope, for the evaluation of the left guttural pouch. The right and left pouches do not communicate with each other. Here the thin septum in the rostral side is artificially transparent to allow endoscope visualization inside left pouch viewed from the right side of the horse.

The guttural pouches are paired, air-filled spaces that extend from the base of the skull and atlas to the nasopharynx[2] (**Fig. 1**). Each pouch communicates with the pharynx through the rostral portion of the respective auditory tube that is 2 to 3 cm long and funnel shaped, opening at the pharyngeal orifice (approximately 3 cm), located at the dorsolateral aspect of the nasopharyngeal lateral wall, known as the ostia[3] (see **Fig. 1**; **Fig. 2**A). These pharyngeal openings are identified as oblique slits lying rostral and ventral to the pharyngeal recess. The medial wall of each opening is composed of a fibrocartilage flap oriented in a rostrodorsal-to-caudoventral direction.[4] Each guttural pouch roof has direct contact with the sphenoid bone, the longus capitis and longus colli muscles, the tympanic bulla, the temporohyoid joint, and the ventral condylar fossa. Laterally, the pouches lie against the medial pterygoid muscle, the digastricus, and the parotid and mandibular salivary glands (see **Figs. 1** and **2**B, C). The medial retropharyngeal lymph nodes are located between the pharynx and ventral wall of the pouch, and they can be identified beneath the guttural pouch membrane on the floor of the medial compartment.[3,5]

The floor of the pouch is adjacent to the dorsal aspect of the nasopharynx, and the caudal extent of the guttural pouch is at the level of the parotid salivary gland.

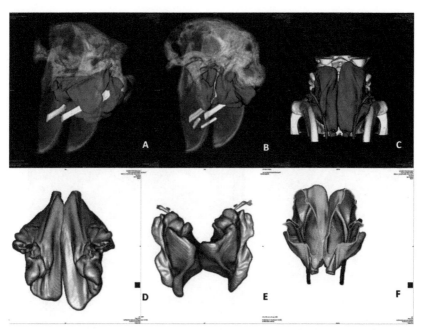

Fig. 2. Guttural pouch CT reconstruction in a healthy 6-month-old Arabian foal. Images were obtained during general anesthetic protocol with 1-mm sections and 3-dimensional software reconstruction. A–C, normal anatomy and position of guttural pouch associated with the foal head and bone structures.(A) note the auditory tube rostral portion. (B), caudal part of the auditory tube enters the tympanic orifice. (C), ventral part (floor) of the 2 pouches showing the medial and lateral compartments and stylohyoid bone (blue). D–F, normal anatomy of an isolated guttural pouch. (D), dorsal view. (E), caudal view. Note the molded stylohyoid sulcus and the auditory tube rostral portion. Note the space between the guttural pounch and skull that is filled by longus capitis and rectus capitis ventralis muscles. (F), dorsal view of a normal guttural pouch without part of the roof showing the left and right structures and lateral and medial compartments separated by a thin septum in the rostral side.

This caudal portion folds over and covers the stylohyoid bone, coursing through its caudolateral aspect and creating an incomplete division that results in a larger medial compartment and a smaller lateral compartment[1,5,6] (see **Figs. 1** and **2**D, E). The caudal portion of the stylohyoid bone articulates with the short tympanohyoid bone, which in turn articulates with the petrous portion of the temporal bone at the skull base. Cranial nerves VII (facial) and VIII (vestibulocochlear) are located in this part of the temporal bone where they are exposed to fractures associated with temporohyoid osteoarthropathy.[5,7] The left and right guttural pouches have nearly the same capacity.[8] The medial compartment is 2 to 3 times the size of the lateral compartment and extends more caudally and ventrally[6,9] (see **Fig. 2**C, D). The right and left pouches do not communicate with each other and are symmetrically separated rostrally by a thin septum and caudally by the longus capitis and rectus capitis ventralis muscles[4,8,10] (**Fig. 2**F).The auricular cartilage is in close contact with the dorsolateral aspect of the guttural pouch. This contact is so intimate that movement of the ear displaces the auricular cartilage on endoscopy.[11] The caudal portion of the auditory tube enters the canal medial to the muscular process of the

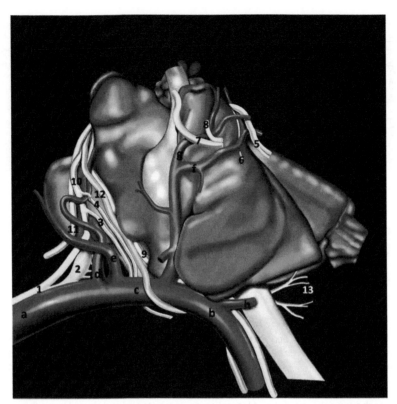

Fig. 3. Nervous structures and arteries with direct association with guttural pouch. 1, vagosympathetic trunk; 2, cranial cervical ganglion; 3, cranial laryngeal nerve; 4, pharyngeal branch of vagus nerve; 5, mandibular nerve; 6, chorda tympani nerve; 7, facial nerve; 8, auriculotemporal nerve; 9, glossopharyngeal nerve; 10, vagus nerve; 11, accessory nerve; 12, hypoglossal nerve; 13, pharyngeal branch of glossopharyngeal nerve. a, common carotid artery; b, linguofacial trunk; c, external carotid artery; d, internal carotid artery; e, occipital artery; f, maxillary artery; g, superficial temporal artery; h, lingual artery.

tympanic part of the temporal bone and enters the tympanic orifice[3,12] (see **Fig. 2**B, E).

Several structures are found adjacent to the equine guttural pouches, including cranial nerves IX (glossopharyngeal), X (vagus), XI (accessory), and XII (hypoglossal); the stylohyoid bone; and the temporohyoid joint. Also in close proximity are cranial nerves V and VII, the cranial cervical ganglion, the cervical sympathetic trunk, the internal carotid artery, and the external carotid artery and its branches (the caudal auricular artery, superficial temporal artery, and maxillary artery).[13] These anatomical structures are depicted in **Fig. 3** and listed in **Table 1**. When affected by guttural pouch disease, these nervous structures may cause a diversity of neurologic signs in addition to epistaxis or abnormal nasal secretions.

The following important structures are located associated with the lateral compartment: the external carotid, superficial temporal and maxillary arteries; the maxillary-facial vein; the facial nerve, and the chorda tympani.[14,15] The external carotid artery travels beside the medial compartment ventral to the stylohyoid bone, along the lateral compartment, where it gives off the caudal auricular and superficial temporal

Table 1
Cranial nerve and sympathetic structures in direct contact with the guttural pouch in the horse

Neural Structure	Brief Description	Innervated Structures	Possible Clinical Signs Associated with Damage and Clinical Investigation
Mandibular nerve (branch of V)	Largest of the three branches of the trigeminal nerve (V). Contains sensory, motor and parasympathetic fibers. Originates the following nerves: a) Motor nerves: masticatory nerve, mylohyoid nerve, medial pterygoid nerve, lateral pterygoid nerve, nerve to tensor veli palatini and nerve to tensor tympani; b) Sensory nerves: buccal nerve, auriculotemporal nerve, lingual nerve and inferior alveolar nerve.	Innervates the major muscles of mastication (temporal and masseter, pterygoids and rostral digastricus), muscle extrinsic to the tongue (mylohyoideus), mucosa of the oral cavity and some salivary glands. The tensor veli palatini tenses the soft palate and retracts the soft palate away from the dorsal pharyngeal wall (this expands the nasopharynx during inspiration) and assists the levator veli palatini (innervated by the glossopharyngeal plexus) by moving the soft palate dorsally to prevent entry of food into the nasopharynx during swallowing. The nerve to the tensor tympani dampens sounds (for example, sounds produced from chewing). The buccal nerve provides sensory innervation to the mucous membranes of the cheek and supplies parasympathetic fibers to the buccal glands. The lingual nerve provides sensory innervation to the rostral two thirds of the tongue and parasympathetic innervations to the sublingual and mandibular salivary glands; the inferior alveolar nerve innervates the inferior teeth and innervates the skin of the inferior lip.	Unilateral lesions of this nerve at the guttural pouch region can cause temporal, masseter, pterygoid and rostral digastricus atrophy (usually after 10 days). Bilateral lesions can cause dropped jaw and an inability to prehend food and mastication. Asymmetrical lesions can cause asymmetrical muscle atrophy and a slightly deviated mandible (more commonly observed weeks later). Decreased sensation in the inferior lip can be observed. No abnormalities will occur at the ophthalmic or maxillary branches at the guttural pouch level (sensory components of the palpebral reflex and face sensitivity are preserved).
Auriculotemporal nerve (branch of mandibular nerve)	It is a sensory branch of the mandibular nerve.	This nerve is sensory and also contains parasympathetic fibers to the parotid gland.	Even if affected after guttural pouch disease, it is clinically difficult to evaluate in horses.

(continued on next page)

Table 1
(continued)

Neural Structure	Brief Description	Innervated Structures	Possible Clinical Signs Associated with Damage and Clinical Investigation
Facial nerve (VII)	The facial nerve has several branches: major petrosal, stapedial, chorda tympani, auricular, auriculopalpebral, buccal, cervical and digastricus.	These different branches are responsible for innervating the muscles related to facial expression: the muscles of the external ear (auricular nerve), the muscles of the external ear and eyelid (auriculopalpebral nerve), the muscles of the superior lip and nose (dorsal buccal branch), the muscles of the cheek and inferior lip (ventral buccal branch) and the caudal portion of digastricus (digastricus branch). It also has sensory components from the skin in the internal surface of external ear, and it contributes to lacrimal gland innervation.	Unilateral lesions result in facial paralysis with a loss of face symmetry due to dropped ear, ptosis (tonus can be tested by elevating the superior eyelid), deviation of the nose and superior lip (toward the normal, innervated side) and flaccid inferior lip. Severe lesions will cause difficulty in food prehension. Lesions may be caused by damage in the petrosal portion of the temporal bone due to fractures associated with temporohyoid osteoarthropathy that affect all branches of the facial nerve. Lesions in this region can also cause differences in tear production; thus, using a Schirmer test can be helpful to compare both sides. These clinical signs can be associated with peripheral vestibular disease due to damage of the vestibular portion of the vestibulocochlear nerve (ipsilateral head tilt; loss of equilibrium and horizontal nystagmus with the rapid phase toward the normal side and positional ventral strabismus). Facial nerve has a close association with the vestibulocochlear nerve in the internal acoustic meatus of the petrosal portion of the temporal bone (this is an important point, as both can be affected in cases of fractures associated with temporohyoid osteoarthropathy). Although not primarily related to a guttural pouch disease, this problem can be evaluated with guttural pouch endoscopy.
Chorda tympani nerve (branch of VII)	It is a branch of the facial nerve. This separation occurs before the facial nerve exits the skull.	Provides sensory gustatory innervations to the cranial two thirds of the tongue and parasympathetic fibers to the mandibular and sublingual salivary glands.	Difficult to evaluate in horses.

(continued on next page)

Table 1
(continued)

Neural Structure	Brief Description	Innervated Structures	Possible Clinical Signs Associated with Damage and Clinical Investigation
Glossopharyngeal nerve (IX)	Has three main branches: pharyngeal, carotid sinus and lingual.	Carries general sensory fibers from the pharynx, the middle ear and the caudal 1/3 of the tongue (lingual). Carries visceral sensory fibers from the carotid bodies (carotid sinus). Supplies parasympathetic fibers to the parotid salivary gland and motor fibers to stylopharyngeus muscle (pharyngeal branch).	Sensory components are difficult to evaluate but can contribute to clinical signs associated with lesions affecting the motor component leading to dysphagia. Observation should be performed during swallowing of food and water. The pharynx should be evaluated with and without an endoscope. The presence of food can be observed in the nostrils of affected horses. Lesions can cause dorsal nasopharyngeal collapse.
Pharyngeal branch of the glossopharyngeal nerve (IX)	Neurons of this branch meet with the pharyngeal branches of the vagus to form the pharyngeal plexus. Neurons from this plexus supply the pharyngeal muscles and mucosa.	Innervates the pharyngeal mucosa (sensory) and the stylopharyngeus muscle (dilator muscle of the pharynx that also contributes to the swallowing process).	Lesions can cause dysphagia and dorsal nasopharyngeal collapse. (Refer to information provided for the IX nerve above).
Vagus nerve (X)	The most important branches are the auricular, pharyngeal, cranial laryngeal, cardiac, recurrent laryngeal nerve, pulmonary branches and vagal trunks to the abdominal viscera. Note that the components of the recurrent laryngeal nerve are within the vagus nerve at the level of the guttural pouch. This nerve itself arises within the cranial mediastinum.	All of the pharyngeal muscles (except the stylopharyngeus) are innervated by the vagus nerve. The laryngeal muscles are innervated by the cranial (cricothyroid muscle) and recurrent laryngeal nerves (other intrinsic laryngeal muscles).	Vagal lesions at the guttural pouch site could affect all branches except the auricular. Dysphagia and inspiratory dyspnea (due to laryngeal paralysis or displacement of the soft palate) are the clinical signs that are observed with vagus lesions at the guttural pouch site. Abnormal sounds (roaring) can be observed during exercise, and this information can be missed during rest in some horses. Endoscopic examination should be performed (swallowing and laryngeal movements).

(continued on next page)

Table 1
(continued)

Neural Structure	Brief Description	Innervated Structures	Possible Clinical Signs Associated with Damage and Clinical Investigation
Pharyngeal branch of the vagus nerve (X)	The most important motor nerve of the pharynx, this nerve branches from the vagus nerve near the cranial cervical ganglion and courses cranioventrally along the medial wall of the guttural pouch to the dorsal wall of the pharynx, where it ramifies in the pharyngeal plexus (association of pharyngeal branch of the vagus nerve and the pharyngeal branch of the glossopharyngeal nerve). From the plexus, branches are distributed to the muscles and mucous membrane of the pharynx (except the stylopharyngeus) and the muscles of the soft palate, except the tensor veli palatini.	Innervates pharyngeal muscles except the stylopharyngeusmuscle and provides sensory innervation for the mucosa of pharynx and larynx. This pharyngeal branch is also responsible for innervating the pterygopharyngeus muscle and levator veli palatini muscle (probably associated with opening mechanisms of the guttural pouch orifice. This mechanism is also related to the action of the stylopharyngeus muscle, which is innervated by the pharyngeal branch of the glossopharyngeal nerve, and the tensor veli palatine, which is innervated by the mandibular nerve). The levator veli palatini muscle elevates the soft palate during swallowing, vocalization,and eructation, and it facilitates oral ventilation. This branch is also important for innervation of the palatopharyngeus and palatinus muscles (their contraction shortens the soft palate and depresses the caudal portion toward the tongue). These muscles associated with tensor veli palatine (innervated by mandibular branch) and levator veli palatini muscles determine the soft palate position.	Dysphagia and dorsal displacement of the soft palate. The action of the levator veli palatini muscle can be evaluated during endoscopic examination of the upper airway when the gag reflex is stimulated.

(continued on next page)

Table 1
(continued)

Neural Structure	Brief Description	Innervated Structures	Possible Clinical Signs Associated with Damage and Clinical Investigation
Cranial laryngeal nerve (branch of X)	Has two components: a sensory internal branch and a motor external branch.	Innervates the laryngeal mucosa cranial to the glottis (contributes to the cough reflex and provides afferent information to the central nervous system, signaling contraction of upper airway muscles to resist dynamic collapse in the upper airway) and is motor to cricothyroid muscle.	Cricothyroid muscle dysfunction may be implicated in vocal fold collapse and likely causes inspiratory airway obstruction in exercising horses. Exercise endoscopic examination and EMG studies can help evaluation. The cranial laryngeal nerve is also important for receiving mechanoreceptor information from the larynx.
Vagosympathetic trunk and cranial cervical ganglion	Contains sympathetic fibers (cervical sympathetic trunk and cranial cervical ganglion) and parasympathetic and visceral sensory vagal nerve fibers (vagosympathetic trunk).	Lesions of guttural pouch structures at this site can cause abnormalities mainly associated with sympathetic fibers located at or near the cranial cervical ganglion, resulting in Horner syndrome. Vagus nerve lesions can affect the fibers that will enter the recurrent laryngeal nerve.	Horner syndrome in horses is characterized by ptosis, hyperthermia and unilateral sudoresis of the face and cranial neck, whereas enophthalmos, third eyelid protrusion and miosis are less obvious signs. Lesions at different sites can cause this syndrome, but guttural pouch endoscopic examination is important to rule out lesions at this site. Laryngeal dysfunction can occur because of lesions of vagal fibers that will enter the recurrent laryngeal nerve and can be evaluated with an endoscopic procedure looking for laryngeal dysfunction.

(continued on next page)

Table 1
(continued)

Neural Structure	Brief Description	Innervated Structures	Possible Clinical Signs Associated with Damage and Clinical Investigation
Accessory nerve (XI)	Has two different branches. The internal branch joins the vagus nerve intracranially before the guttural pouch region and will contribute to the formation of the RLN. The external branch is formed by the spinal roots and contains motor fibers to neck muscles.	The external branch innervates the trapezius, sternocephalicus and cleidocephalicus muscles.	Cranial nerve XI lesions at the level of the guttural pouch can affect only the external branch of the accessory nerve. During examination, the atrophy of neck muscles should be looked for, which is usually not present. EMG studies can help. To affect the internal branch fibers, a vagus nerve lesion must be present at the guttural pouch level. In this case, laryngeal endoscopy would be helpful.
Hypoglossal nerve (XII)		Motor innervation to all intrinsic and extrinsic muscles of the tongue (styloglossus, hyoglossus, and genioglossus) as well as the hyoepiglotticus, geniohyoideus, and thyrohyoideus muscles. The hyoepiglotticus muscle attaches the base of the epiglottis to the hyoid bone, and when it contracts, it pulls the epiglottis ventrally toward the base of the tongue, further expanding the nasopharynx. The geniohyoideus (also moves the hyoid bone rostrally) and genioglossus, which are associated with other muscles, increase the lateral and ventral dimensions of the nasopharynx.	Lesions will cause abnormal tongue function. Close inspection is necessary to evaluate symmetry, tonus, movements, deviation, or atrophy. Severe abnormalities can cause dysphagia.

Data from Refs. [2,5,12,33,34,37–42]

arteries and continues as the maxillary artery along the lateral dorsal wall of the lateral compartment[4] (see **Fig. 3**). The maxillary vein can be seen lateral to and slightly deep to the external carotid artery.[5]

The internal carotid artery (ICA) runs from ventral to dorsal along the middle portion of the medial compartment and forms a sigmoid flexure just before reaching the dorsal limit of the pouch. Cranial nerves IX, X, XI, and XII course ventrally along the medial compartment of the guttural pouch and are enveloped in a thin fold of mucosa. These nerves and the sympathetic trunk are intimately associated with the ICA for much of their course within the pouch. The pharyngeal branch of the vagus nerve (X) runs along the floor of the medial compartment before joining the pharyngeal plexus[16] (**Figs. 4** and **5**).

The facial nerve and its branches, as well as the mandibular nerve, pass adjacent to the roof of the guttural pouch.[17] The facial nerve runs dorsally along the lateral recess for approximately 3 to 4 cm and then runs between the mandibular and parotid glands. The mandibular nerve runs along the roof of the lateral recess and then continues on the rostral side of the guttural pouch[8] (see **Fig. 3**). Cranial nerve XII runs caudally between the guttural pouch and atlanto-occipital joint capsule for a distance of approximately 2 cm, passes between the vagus and accessory nerves, turns ventrorostrally, and continues above the pharynx, parallel to the stylohyoid bone and caudal to the linguofacial trunk. Cranial nerve IX turns ventrorostrally over the guttural pouch caudal to the thyrohyoid bone; at that point it is deeper than the external carotid artery and gives off the pharyngeal and lingual branches. Cranial nerve X passes caudally and ventrally, together with the accessory nerve, through a fold of the guttural pouch. These nerves then separate, which allows the hypoglossal nerve to pass between them. The vagus nerve passes ventrally adjacent to the internal carotid artery and crosses the medial aspect of the origin of the occipital artery; its pharyngeal branch crosses the internal carotid artery and runs ventrocranially from the guttural pouch to the dorsal wall of the pharynx[18] (see **Fig. 3**). The pharyngeal branch of cranial nerve X is given off near the cranial cervical ganglion and can be seen as it runs rostroventrally along the guttural pouch toward the wall of the dorsal pharynx, where it ramifies with the pharyngeal branch of IX in the pharyngeal plexus. The pharyngeal branch of IX can be identified as it runs rostrally across the ventral aspect of the stylohyoid bone[5] (see **Figs. 4** and **5**).

GUTTURAL POUCH FUNCTION, EXAMINATION, AND MAIN ABNORMALITIES

Currently, there remains a high level of interest in studies concerning guttural pouch function. Therefore, research has been conducted in order to elucidate and present evidences on the physiologic importance of these structures.[5,7,9,19–22]

Clinical evaluation of the guttural pouch begins with clinical history, patient identification, and inspection followed by external palpation of the structure. The guttural pouches can be assessed by complementary exams such as radiography, ultrasound, and endoscopy.[23] Endoscopy is the exam that most effectively facilitates data collection in cases of guttural pouch disease because it allows direct visualization of the structures of interest.[11] During guttural pouch examinations, exudate, blood, and intraluminal and extraluminal masses may be noted. Bacterial infection or fluid draining from the retropharyngeal lymph nodes may lead to the accumulation of a purulent exudate in the guttural pouches. Intraluminal masses are usually associated with the presence of chondroids or neoplasias such as melanoma, squamous cell carcinoma, hemangiosarcoma, and fibroma.[11] Several authors have provided detailed methods for endoscopy of the guttural pouch, specifically focusing on the introduction of the endoscope into the pouch and photography to assist in anatomical

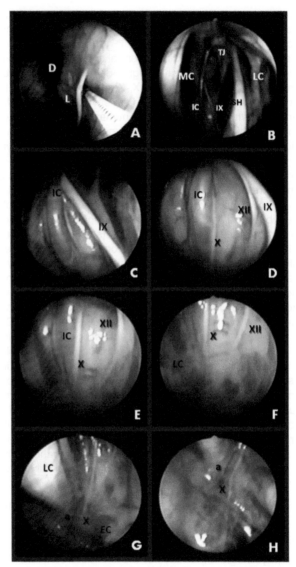

Fig. 4. Left guttural pouch endoscopy in a clinically normal horse. *A* and *B*: D, dorsal pharyngeal recess; L, nasopharyngeal opening of the left guttural pouch; MC, medial compartment; LC, lateral compartment; TJ, temporohyoid joint; SH, stylohyoid bone; IC, internal carotid artery; IX, cranial nerve IX. *C* and *D*: IC, internal carotid artery; IX, cranial nerve IX; XII, cranial nerve XII; X, cranial nerve X. *E* and *F*, LC, longus capitis muscle; IC, internal carotid artery; X, cranial nerve X; XII, cranial nerve XII. *G* and *H*: ventral aspect of the left guttural pouch medial compartment. LC, Longus capitis muscle; EC, external carotid artery; X, cranial nerve X; a, pharyngeal branch of the vagus nerve.

identification.[5,11] Note that the endoscopic examination of patients with epistaxis and suspicious for guttural pouch mycosis must be carefully conducted; clot displacement can occur and ultimately result in fatal hemorrhage.[24] Endoscopic examination is a very useful method to evaluate temporohyoid articulation in horses with peripheral

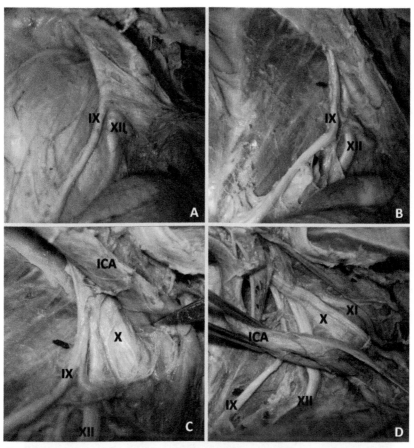

Fig. 5. Cranial nerves postmortem anatomical study (*A, B*). It is possible to observe cranial nerves IX, X, XI, and XII and internal carotid artery (ICA). (*C, D*) Cranial nerves IX, X, XI, and XII course ventrally along the medial compartment of the guttural pouch and are enveloped in a thin fold of mucosa. These nerves are intimately associated with the ICA.

vestibular signs or facial nerve deficits (**Figs. 6–8**). Movement of the temporohyoid articulation can be assessed by simultaneously pushing upward on the lingual process of the basihyoid in the intermandibular space while visualizing the articulation endoscopically. Radiographs can also reveal relevant information because the air-filled guttural pouches provide an ideal contrast medium for radiographic imaging. Lateral projections provide information about the dimensions and content of the guttural pouches.[15] Dorsoventral and ventrodorsal views are used to assess the stylohyoid bone. Radiographs also allow presurgical evaluation and make it possible to accurately locate vascular structures.[25] More recently, computed tomography (CT) and magnetic resonance imaging (MRI) of the guttural pouches have permitted a better understanding of its anatomy and have become important in the diagnosis of tumors or abnormal morphology.[10,26] CT may be most beneficial for imaging of the stylohyoid bone, inner ear, and the petrous portion of the temporal bone in cases of stylohyoid osteoarthropathy.[11,27] Other indirect

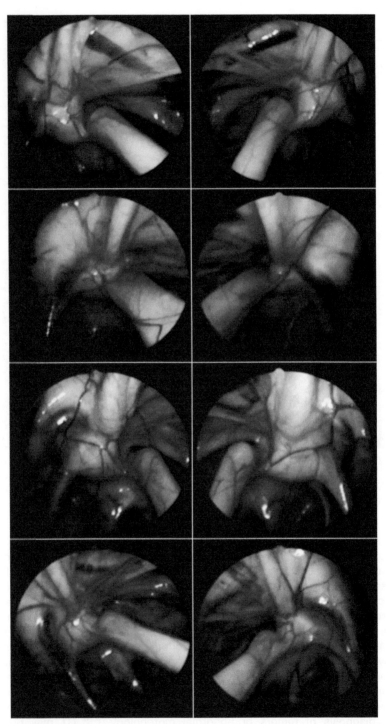

Fig. 6. Endoscopic evaluation of the stylohyoid bone in 4 clinically normal horses showing different anatomic conformation of this region (left and right side).

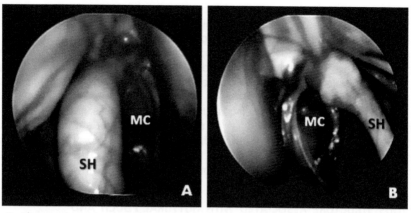

Fig. 7. Abnormal stylohyoid bone conformation in horses with vestibular peripheral syndrome. *A*, right guttural pouch: proliferation of the proximal stylohyoid bone (SH). MC, medial compartment. *B*, Left guttural pouch: proliferation of the proximal SH.

evaluation techniques allow material collection from the guttural pouches for cellular and microbiological analysis.[28]

The major diseases of the guttural pouch are empyema, tympany, and mycosis. Guttural pouch mycosis and longus capitis avulsion are the most common conditions associated with guttural pouch hemorrhage. Other afflictions, including trauma, cysts, and neoplasia, are infrequently encountered.[29] Guttural pouch empyema is the most common disease of the guttural pouch and is defined as the presence of purulent material and chondroids within one or both guttural pouches.[5,11] The most common clinical sign associated with empyema is profuse, unilateral, purulent secretion.[30] Lateral radiographic examination of the region demonstrates fluid lines or concretions inside the pouch.[31] Tympany is a nonpainful distention of the guttural pouch with air, and this disease may be accompanied by fluid accumulation and may also produce external swelling in the parotid region.[7,24] Guttural pouch mycosis is characterized by

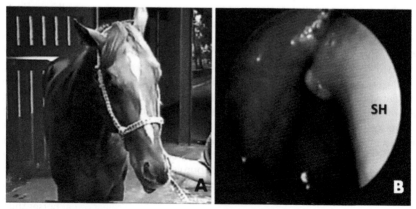

Fig. 8. (*A*) Horse presenting right head tilt and facial paralysis. (*B*) Right guttural pouch stylohyoid osteoarthropathy endoscopic view. SH, stylohyoid bone.

development of fungal plaques on the mucosal walls of the guttural pouches, and it is the disease most associated with cranial nerve abnormalities. The plaques are usually located on the roof of the medial compartment.[24] The most common clinical sign of guttural pouch mycosis is severe epistaxis caused by erosion of the internal carotid artery, external carotid artery, and/or maxillary artery. Other clinical signs include mucopurulent or hemorrhagic nasal discharge, coughing, dysphagia, and a variety of neurologic signs.[5,7,11,24]

There are reviews available that discuss the etiology, diagnosis, and treatment of all of the aforementioned diseases.[6,7,11,15] In summary, it is important to state that the main clinical signs noted with guttural pouch diseases depend on the pathologic process, but the most frequent findings are distension (tympany), mucopurulent discharge (empyema), and epistaxis with or without dysphagia (mycosis).

CONSIDERATIONS ABOUT THE FUNCTION AND IMPORTANCE OF EACH NERVOUS STRUCTURE ASSOCIATED WITH GUTTURAL POUCH AND NEUROLOGIC EVALUATION

The neurologic evaluation in horses has been described in detail previously.[32–36] A logical approach is important and includes the following steps: confirm the presence of neurologic abnormalities, localize the lesion, and determine the nature of the lesions. This process will help to determine a list of differential diagnoses and suggest complementary tests. The importance and function of the nerves and sympathetic structures that are anatomically associated with the guttural pouches are summarized in **Table 1**.

Guttural pouch disease is not a common performance-limiting upper respiratory disorder. However, the cranial nerves that are adjacent to the guttural pouch can become damaged as a result of guttural pouch disease and may cause dysfunction of the muscles they innervate.[43] The major clinical abnormalities due to cranial nerve dysfunction or damage to sympathetic structures that require guttural pouch examination are as follows: dysphagia, Horner syndrome, soft palate displacement, masseter atrophy, facial paralysis (dropped ears and lips, abnormal palpebral reflex, and nose deviation), laryngeal paralysis, abnormal sounds during exercise, peripheral vestibular signs (head tilt, nystagmus, vestibular ataxia, and positional ventral strabismus), and head shaking. It is notable that these abnormalities may have origins other than guttural pouch disease. Thus, guttural pouches are not always responsible for the observed clinical signs. For example, there are numerous causes of dysphagia, of which some have no direct relation to the nervous system, whereas others originate within the central nervous system.[44] For example, Horner syndrome can be caused by interruptions in different regions of the sympathetic pathway (eg, from a cranial thoracic tumor or incorrect administration of a medication in the cervical region).[45,46] Injury to the sympathetic nerve anywhere along the jugular furrow or within the guttural pouch will generally cause sweating on the head and neck caudal to C2 on the ipsilateral side. Soft palate displacement can be caused by an increase in lymph node volume adjacent to guttural pouches. Such discrimination is important and has to be performed for all of the detected abnormalities before considering the guttural pouch as the focus of lesion, especially when other signs of guttural pouch disease are not present. The probability of guttural pouch involvement in any of these pathologic entities highly increases when purulent discharge, bloody mucoid discharge, or any other anomaly is found during inspection. It is also important to note that several reports have described guttural pouch disorders, such as mycosis, neoplasia, or inflammatory processes that did not cause cranial nerve abnormalities because nervous structures were not directly affected.[47–50]

It is important to highlight that some of the nervous structures presented in **Table 1** play an essential role in the movement of the larynx, palate position, and swallowing. The association between guttural pouch diseases (especially guttural pouch mycosis) and normal larynx movements or palate function was previously considered a long time ago,[51] and the comprehension of the importance of the contribution of each cranial nerve for the normal physiologic functions in the horse is still under research.

One area of recent interest is the innervation of muscles responsible for maintaining the function of the larynx and nasopharynx. Branches of the trigeminal, glossopharyngeal, vagus, and hypoglossal nerves supply efferent innervation to the muscles that dilate and constrict the nasopharynx. Most of these nerves, with the exception of the recurrent laryngeal nerves, course adjacent to the guttural pouch and are vulnerable to damage if the guttural pouch becomes inflamed or infected.[37]

The soft palate position is mediated by the correct function of the following muscles: the *tensor veli palatini,* the *levator veli palatini,* the *palatinus* and the *palatopharyngeus* muscles.[39,52] The palatinus and palatopharyngeus muscles are believed to be important in maintaining normal soft palate positioning during breathing and particularly during intense exercise.[53,54] Some clinical disorders can be directly associated with the guttural pouch and its related structures. For example, the hypothesis that dorsal displacement of the soft palate (DDSP) may be caused by dysfunction of the neuromuscular regulation of the soft palate, and this dysfunction may involve the pharyngeal branch of the vagus nerve. The pharyngeal branch of the vagus nerve is intimately associated with the guttural pouch wall and is near the retropharyngeal lymph node. Therefore, lymphadenopathy, inflammation, and infection may damage this branch and cause DDSP.[37] Previous experiments revealed that bilateral blockade of the pharyngeal branch of the vagus nerve from inside the medial compartment of the guttural pouch as it courses across the *longus capitus* muscle caused persistent DDSP in horses.[39] The horses were dysphagic during the blockade experiment, which was likely due to paralysis of the pharyngeal constrictor muscles that are also innervated by the pharyngeal branch of the vagus nerve. Therefore, it is also important to rule out guttural pouch diseases in dysphagic horses. The same authors examined the guttural pouches of all horses presenting with clinical DDSP. There was evidence of guttural pouch inflammation and retropharyngeal lymphadenopathy in many of these horses.[39] A recently published review paper noted that this model, however, did not fully mimic the clinical presentation of DDSP because the experimentally induced DDSP was persistent (ie, it was present at rest as opposed to only developing during exercise). Additionally, the horses also exhibited dysphagia, which is not seen in clinical cases of intermittent DDSP.[54] Based on this information, there was convincing evidence to suggest that neuromuscular dysfunction, including that of the pharyngeal branch of the vagus nerve, palatinus muscle, and palatopharyngeus muscle, might be involved in the pathogenesis of intermittent, dorsal displacement of the soft palate in exercising horses.[5]

Several reports describe the importance of the guttural pouch and related structures for exercise and nasopharyngeal stability, and the hypoglossal nerve also innervates important structures associated with the nasopharynx. One example is the hypoepiglotticus muscle, which exhibits significant activity during inspiration[55] and plays an important role in expanding the nasopharynx.[37] In an experimental study, blockade of the hypoglossal nerve produced an expiratory obstruction similar to that seen in naturally occurring DDSP, with reduced inspiratory and expiratory pharyngeal pressure and increased expiratory tracheal pressure. These data suggest that the stability of the equine upper airway during exercise may be maintained through the hypoglossal nerve.[42] A previous study evaluated the role of the hypoglossal nerve in airway stability in the horse.[56] This study induced hypoglossal dysfunction at the level of the guttural pouch and produced epiglottic retroversion with inspiratory obstruction.[56] As a result, it was not possible to assess the effect on nasopharyngeal stability.

Bilateral glossopharyngeal nerve anaesthesia produced stylopharyngeus muscle dysfunction, dorsal pharyngeal collapse and airway obstruction in horses.[57] It is interesting to note that no signs of dysphagia were observed after bilateral glossopharyngeal nerve anesthesia from inside the guttural pouch.[40,57] It was concluded that glossopharyngeal nerve function may not be essential for normal swallowing function in otherwise healthy horses.[40] Dysphagia associated with guttural pouch disease, therefore, is mostly due to injury of the vagus nerve.

The neurologic evaluation of a horse with suspected abnormal laryngeal function should include a complete neurologic examination because left-sided recurrent laryngeal neuropathy may occur in conjunction with other neurologic signs. These signs rarely relate to brain or spinal cord lesions. Although the recurrent laryngeal nerve arises as a branch of the vagus nerve in the cranial thorax, these axons are a component of the vagus nerve from the level of the foramen lacerum to the cranial thorax. Laryngeal paralysis may be associated with dysphagia when a lesion affects the vagus nerve prior to the origin of its pharyngeal branch. Cervical lesions that affect the vagosympathetic trunk may cause laryngeal paralysis along with Horner syndrome. The latter may include sweating over the ipsilateral side of the head and cranial neck area.[58]

NEUROLOGIC ABNORMALITIES ASSOCIATED WITH GUTTURAL POUCH DISEASE

Several reports have presented data on neurologic abnormalities as a consequence of guttural pouch disease, corroborating the importance of guttural pouch evaluation in equine neurologic disease cases. Mycosis of the guttural pouch is one of the most frequent and the most important abnormality associated with reports on the concomitant disturbance of cranial nerves. Non–exercise-associated, moderate-to-severe epistaxis is the most common clinical sign and is a consequence of fungal erosion of the internal carotid artery, external carotid, or maxillary artery walls. The second most common presenting sign is dysphagia, which follows damage to the pharyngeal branches of the glossopharyngeal and vagus nerves.[59] Pharyngeal paralysis is the most frequent neuropathy that accompanies guttural pouch mycosis in the horse, followed by laryngeal hemiplegia.[60] These characteristics were also observed in the following descriptions of guttural pouch mycosis in horses.

A previously published study reported 32 cases of guttural pouch mycosis describing that dysphagia was observed in 17 horses, Horner syndrome in 4 cases, and facial paralysis in 1 case.[47] The postmortem study revealed that the close proximity of the glossopharyngeal, vagus, and accessory nerves to the lesion sometimes led to their involvement in the disease. This involvement varied in severity from slight swelling of the myelin sheaths and Schwann cells and dilation of the intraneural capillaries to heavy leukocytic infiltration and necrosis associated with fungal penetration of fibers. In addition, chromatolysis, degenerative swelling, and vacuolation of neurons in the cranial cervical ganglion were observed. These lesions explain the observation of laryngeal and pharyngeal hemiplegia and the Horner syndrome. The degree of damage to the glossopharyngeal, vagus, and accessory nerves varied, and microscopically there was mild, degenerative swelling of nerve fibers in animals that did not show previous nervous signs. Other horses had severe neuritis that did not allow a return to normal function.[61]

A horse was diagnosed with guttural pouch mycosis (presenting with swelling in the laryngeal region and nasal discharge), and later dysphagia was observed.[62] Dysphagia developed in a 2-year-old Quarter Horse filly following an incident in which she fell over backward while exercising on a mechanical horse walker. Hyperextension of the neck at this time apparently caused unilateral rupture of the *longus capitis, rectus capitis ventralis major,* and *rectus capitis ventralis minor* muscles at their insertions. An existing mycotic lesion involving the dorsomedial wall of the left guttural pouch may have weakened the insertion point of the involved muscles. Tearing of the tendinous insertion of these muscles caused damage to cranial nerves IX, X, and XI and the left guttural pouch, with subsequent development of mild transitory epistaxis, laryngeal hemiplegia, pharyngeal paralysis, and dysphagia.[63] Additional guttural pouch mycosis cases that resulted in neurologic signs and are described in the literature are reviewed in **Table 2**.

Empyema is the most common guttural pouch disease and can result in pharyngeal and/or laryngeal dysfunction.[43] Dysphagia due to cranial nerve damage was previously reported in a horse with bilateral guttural pouch empyema.[77] Chronic empyema with associated signs of cranial nerve involvement, such as dysphagia or laryngeal hemiplegia, was also described.[11]

Another report described 3 cases of hemorrhage into the guttural pouch associated with a rupture of the *longus capitis* muscle, not associated with mycosis, empyema, neoplasia, or foreign bodies. The source of the hemorrhage appeared to be a rupture of the *longus capitis* muscle and its associated vascular supply. The authors did not observe cranial nerve deficits in these horses.[50]

Guttural pouch tympany was described in 15 cases, and only 1 presented with dysphagia. Although the cause of dysphagia was not investigated, it was tentatively attributed to mechanical interference with normal pharyngeal function rather than cranial nerve damage.[78] Guttural pouch tympany does not seem to be a cause of cranial nerve problems in foals, and a retrospective study of 50 cases did not reveal cranial nerve involvement.[79]

Guttural pouch neoplasias, which are mostly melanomas and hemangiosarcomas, are infrequently described. Guttural pouch neoplasias associated with cranial nerve deficits are especially uncommon; nevertheless, dysphagia was described in a horse diagnosed with a guttural pouch hemangioma located on the medial compartment roof of the left guttural pouch.[80] Three horses were diagnosed with guttural pouch neoplasia, of which one had a hemangiosarcoma invading the guttural pouch and several other tissues. This horse presented with neurologic signs (eg, dropped lower lip and decreased reflex movements of the epiglottis).[81]

GUTTURAL POUCH DISEASE MAY AFFECT SURROUNDING STRUCTURES AND CAUSE NEUROLOGIC PROBLEMS

The anatomy of the guttural pouch and its position inside the head, which is near important structures such as the ear, skull, and atlas, can result in damage because lesions can eventually jeopardize contiguous areas and cause neurologic abnormalities. Some examples of vision-related structural abnormalities, encephalitis, or bone abnormalities are noted in the literature and highlight the importance of guttural pouch evaluation for differential diagnosis. Recurrent epistaxis, in addition to locomotor and visual disturbances leading to blindness in a 7-year-old gelding, appeared to have resulted from a spreading fungal granuloma of the guttural pouch. The inflamed area extended to the intracranial segment of the right optic nerve and to the region adjacent to the optic chiasm.[82] A horse with a head tilt and secretions in the left external acoustic meatus, which was associated with bilateral squamous cell carcinoma of the guttural pouch and left middle ear, was also previously reported.[83] Acute vestibular disease resulting from extension of an *Aspergillus* guttural pouch infection

Table 2
Brief summary including reports describing guttural pouch mycosis associated with neurologic signs

Author and Year	Case Study	Clinical Signs	Nervous Structures Affected (author's observation)	Observations
Björklund and Palsson, (1970)[64]	Seven cases of guttural pouch mycosis	Three horses presented dysphagia and 1 horse presented with facial paralysis.		The horse with facial paralysis had the two-thirds of the roof and the septum between the pouches affected. Facial nerve degeneration was noted.
Rawlinson and Jones, (1978)[65]	Two horses	Both presented with dysphagia, and one had ipsilateral laryngeal hemiplegia.		
Dixon et al, (1981)[66]	One horse	Dysphagia, left arytenoids with reduced movement and left sternocephalicus muscle atrophy.	Paralysis in cranial nerves IX, X, and XI and cranial cervical ganglion.	Middle and external ear infection were also observed.
Hilbert et al, (1981)[67]	One horse	Pharyngeal, soft palate, laryngeal, and facial paralysis. The horse was unable to vocalize normally.	Histologically, there were numerous nerve fascicles with severe degenerative changes.	Although the lesion probably affected the facial nerve over the lateral aspect of the guttural pouch, the auriculopalpebral branch was not affected because ear drooping was not observed.
Lane and Mair, (1987)[68]	Review paper	Guttural pouch mycosis is a possible cause of headshaking in horses.		

(continued on next page)

Table 2
(continued)

Author and Year	Case Study	Clinical Signs	Nervous Structures Affected (author's observation)	Observations
Greet, (1987)[69]	35 cases of guttural pouch mycosis	Eleven horses presented 1 or more signs related to cranial nerve dysfunction (9 cases with dysphagia, 1 case with tongue paralysis, 1 case with facial paralysis, 4 cases with laryngeal paralysis, and 1 horse presenting with Horner syndrome).		
Walmsley, (1988)[70]	One horse	A dysphagic horse that also presented with a stiff neck.		Atlanto-occipital arthropathy was present.
Howarth and Lane, (1990)[71]	Three horses	Dysphagia with a bilateral nasal discharge in all 3. One horse also presented with facial paralysis, sternocephalicus muscle atrophy, collapse of the left dorsal pharyngeal wall, and left laryngeal hemiplegia. The second horse presented with Horner syndrome, laryngeal hemiplegia, and reduced pharyngeal constrictor activity. The third horse was diagnosed with dysphagia due to pharyngeal hemiplegia.		

(continued on next page)

Table 2
(continued)

Author and Year	Case Study	Clinical Signs	Nervous Structures Affected (author's observation)	Observations
Kipar and Frese, (1993)[72]	Two cases	Both presented with dysphagia and severe atrophy of the lingual muscles (lingual hemiplegia), and one of them also showed signs of head shaking.	Signs were due to hypoglossal neuritis.	Necrotizing and purulent neuritis of the hypoglossal nerve with fungal hyphae extending between myelinated nerve fibers were found.
Dixon et al, (2001)[73]	Retrospective study of 375 horses with laryngeal paralysis	Seven cases were caused by guttural pouch mycosis. Of these cases, 5 presented with dysphagia, 4 presented with right laryngeal paralysis, and 3 were affected on the left side. One horse also presented with facial paralysis, and one presented with Horner syndrome.		
Cabañes et al, (2003)[74]	One horse	Dysphagia, DDSP, and laryngeal hemiplegia		
Laugier et al, (2009)[75]	Retrospective study using a necropsy survey of neurologic diseases	Seven cases (1.3% of the total 543 cases studied) of polyneuritis were associated with guttural pouch mycosis.		
Laus et al, (2010)[76]	One donkey	Dysphagia	Damage to cranial nerves IX, X, XI, and XII	

to the stylohyoid and petrous portion of the temporal bone has also been documented.[84,85] A horse with erosion of the atlanto-occipital joint capsule at a point in direct contact with a guttural pouch affected by mycotic infection was described as well. This horse presented with a stiff neck, and the authors also associated the guttural pouch mycosis with a middle and external ear infection.[66] A similar problem was described in a horse with atlanto-occipital arthropathy following guttural pouch mycosis.[70] Mycotic encephalitis in a horse with guttural pouch mycosis was diagnosed, and in this case, the authors suggested that brain involvement occurred after hematogenous spreading from the primary site. The authors noted that many small vessels in the guttural pouch mucosa and underlying tissues were thrombosed and invaded by fungal elements, thus providing access to the vascular system.[86] A similar complication was also previously observed.[87]

NEUROLOGIC COMPLICATIONS ASSOCIATED WITH GUTTURAL POUCH TREATMENTS

The techniques for surgical correction of guttural pouch abnormalities, the difficulty in identifying nervous structures in a severely inflamed pouch with compromised anatomy, and the difficulty in identifying vascular structures in normal horses or in those with aberrant branches can lead to complications. Some of these complications may be neurologic in character.[7,88,89] The literature reports a number of neurologic abnormalities after surgical procedures for tympany or empyema or for the treatment of guttural pouch mycosis.[78,90] Surgical correction for bilateral guttural tympany in a foal resulted in postoperative pharyngeal neuromuscular dysfunction and a flaccid tongue due mainly to glossopharyngeal and hypoglossal nerve damage and possible injury to the accessory and pharyngeal branch of the vagus nerve.[91] The treatment of guttural pouch mycosis using vascular occlusion procedures is critical for the management of this disease but can result in different types of nervous structure abnormalities by direct or indirect damage due to abnormal blood flow, especially to the eye.[92] Ischemic optic neuropathy accompanied by blindness after surgical occlusion of the external and internal carotid and greater palatine arteries, performed as part of the management of guttural pouch mycosis, was reported in a horse.[90,93] Blindness was explained as a steal phenomenon that can occur when a major artery is occluded and the blood is diverted by backflow from collateral channels into the segment distal to the occlusion. This phenomenon can drain off or steal a considerable amount of flow from the external ophthalmic artery (the major blood supply to the horse eye).[92,93] A complete review that describes complications due to the surgical treatment of guttural pouch diseases was recently published.[92] The infusion of irritating substances into the guttural pouch is known to produce neurologic disease. Caustic solutions such as alcohol/iodine products should never be infused into the pouch.

SUMMARY

The close relationship between guttural pouches, cranial nerves, and sympathetic structures make neurologic abnormalities due to diseases of the guttural pouches (especially mycosis) possible. Recognition of epistaxis or mucopurulent nasal discharge, together with signs of dysfunction of the cranial nerves in contact with the guttural pouches, are important key points in order to consider a comprehensive evaluation of these structures and further definitive diagnosis. Diseases of the guttural pouches can also cause signs such as dysphagia, abnormal soft palate positioning, laryngeal paralysis, and Horner syndrome due to lesions in one or more of the cranial nerves or sympathetic structures involved with these functions. Therefore, an accurate diagnosis is essential for treatment.

ACKNOWLEDGMENTS

The authors thank Dr Alexander de Lahunta for critical review of **Figs. 1** and **3** and **Table 1** and for considerations about the text; Dr Thalita Machado for preparing **Figs. 5** and **6**; Dr José Ricardo de Carvalho Pinto e Silva for providing technical assistance during postmortem guttural pouch anatomical study; Drs Mariana Palumbo and Diego Delfiol for reviewing the reference list; Dr Vania Maria de Vasconcelos Machado for the guttural pouch CT procedure; Mr Heraldo André Catalan Rosa for technical assistance during guttural pouch CT procedure and 3-dimensional reconstruction; Dr Iriam Gomes Starling (medical illustrator) for preparing **Figs. 1** and **3**; and Dr Armen Thomassian for performing endoscopic examination of the horse presented at **Fig. 8**.

REFERENCES

1. Dyce KM, Wolfgang WO, Wensing CJG. The head and ventral neck of the horse. In: Textbook of veterinary anatomy. 4th edition. St Louis (MO): Saunders Elsevier; 2009. p. 501–32.
2. Budras KD, Sack WO, Röck S. Head. In: Anatomy of the horse. 5th edition. Hannover (Germany): Schluetersche; 2010. p. 32–51.
3. de Lahunta A, Habel RE. Hear, horn. In: Applied veterinary anatomy. 1st edition. Philadelphia: WB Saunders; 1986. p. 55–65.
4. Pleasant DB, Berry DB II. Disorders of guttural pouch. In: Robinson NE, Sprayberry KA. Current therapy in equine medicine. 6th edition. St Louis (MO): Saunders Elsevier; 2009. p. 250–4.
5. Holcombe SJ, Ducharme NG. Upper airway function of normal horses during exercise. In: Hinchcliff KW, Kaneps AJ, Geor RJ, editors. Equine sports medicine and surgery: basic and clinical sciences of the equine athlete. Philadelphia: Saunders; 2004. p. 553–6.
6. Edwards GB, Greet T. Disorders of the guttural pouches (auditory diverticuli). In: McGorum DC, Dixon PM, Robinson NE, editors. Equine respiratory medicine and surgery. 1st edition. Philadelphia: Elsevier Saunders; 2007. p. 419–36.
7. Freeman DE, Hardy J. Guttural pouch. In: Auer JA, Stick JA, editors. Equine surgery. 3rd edition. St Louis (MO): Saunders Elsevier; 2006. p. 591–607.
8. Manglai D, Wada R, Endo H, et al. Macroscopic anatomy of the auditory tube diverticulum (guttural pouch) in the Thoroughbred equine: a silicon mold approach. Okajimas Folia Anat Jpn 2000;76:335–6.
9. Barber SM. Disease of the guttural pouches. In: Colahan PT, Merritt AM, Moore JN, et al, editors. Equine medicine and surgery. St Louis (MO): Mosby; 1999. p. 501–12.
10. Oto C, Haziroglu RM. Magnetic resonance imaging of the guttural pouch (*diverticulum tubae auditivae*) and its related structures in donkey (*Equus asinus*). Ankara U'niv Vet Fak Derg 2011;58:1–4.
11. Hardy J, Léveillé R. Diseases of guttural pouches. Vet Clin Equine 2003;19:123–58.
12. Sisson S. Equine myology. In: Sisson S, Grossman JD, Getty R, editors. The anatomy of domestic animals. 5th edition. Philadelphia: WB Saunders; 1975. p. 386–7.
13. Polloch PJ. Diagnosis and management of guttural pouch mycosis. Equine Vet Educ 2007;19:522–7.
14. Freeman DE. Diagnosis and treatment of diseases of the guttural pouch (part I). Compend Contin Educ Pract Vet 1980;(Suppl 1):3–11.

15. Perkins GA, Pease A, Crotty E, et al. Diagnosing guttural pouch disorders and managing guttural pouch empyema in adult horses. Cornell Univ Compend Contin Educ 2003;25:966–83.

16. Barakzai S. In: Handbook of equine respiratory endoscopy. 1st edition. New York: Saunders Elsevier; 2007. p. 135.

17. König HE, Budras KD, Seeger JS, et al. Zur topographisch-klinischen Anatomie des Luftsackes (Diverticulum tubae auditivae) beim Pferd. Pferdeheilkunde 2010;26: 152–6.

18. Godinho HP, Getty R. Nervos cranianos. In: Getty R, editor. Anatomia dos animais domésticos. 5th edition. Rio de Janeiro (Brazil): Guanabara Koogan; 1986. p. 608–20.

19. Hawkins DL. Diseases of guttural pouches. In. Robinson NE, editor. Current therapy in equines. 3rd edition. St Louis (MO): Saunders; 1992. p. 275–80.

20. Baptiste KE. A preliminary study on the role of the equine guttural pouches in selective brain cooling. Vet J 1998;155:139–48.

21. Baptiste KE, Naylor JM, Bailey J, et al. A function for guttural pouches in the horse. Nature 2000;403:382–3.

22. Mitchell G, Fuller A, Maloney SK, et al. Guttural pouches, brain temperature and exercise in horses. Biol Lett 2006;2:475–7.

23. Chiesa OA, Lopez C, Domingo M, et al. A percutaneous technique for guttural pouch lavage. Equine Pract 2000;22:8–11.

24. Ainsworth DM, Hackett RP. Disorders of the respiratory system. In: Reed SM, Bayly WM, Sellon DC, editors. Equine internal medicine. 2nd edition. St Louis (MO): Saunders; 2004. p. 289–354.

25. MacDonald DG, Fretz PB, Baptiste KE, et al. Anatomic, radiographic and physiologic comparisons of the internal carotid and maxillary artery in the horse. Vet J 1999;158: 182–9.

26. Sasaki M, Hayashi Y, Koie H. CT Examinations of the guttural pouch (auditory tube diverticulum) in Prezwalski's horse (Equus przewalskii). J Vet Med Sci 1999;61: 1019–22.

27. Hilton H, Puchalski SM, Aleman M. The computed tomographic appearance of equine temporohyoid osteoarthropathy. Vet Radiol Ultrasound 2009;50:151–6.

28. Chiesa OA, Vidal D, Domingo M, et al. Cytological and bacteriological findings in guttural pouch lavages of clinically normal horses. Vet Rec 1999;144:346–9.

29. Scarratt WK, Crisman MV. Neoplasia of the respiratory tract. Vet Clin North Am Equine Pract 1998;14:451–73.

30. Carmalt J. Guttural pouch diseases in the horse. Large Anim Vet Rounds 2002;2:1–6.

31. Lepage OM. Disorders of the guttural pouches. In: Lekeux P, editor. Equine respiratory diseases. Available at: www.ivis.org.

32. Lunn DP, Mayhew IG. The neurological evaluation of horses. Equine Vet Educ 1989;94–101.

33. de Lahunta A, Glass E. The neurologic examination. In: de Lahunta A, Glass E, editors. Veterinary neuroanatomy and clinical neurology. 3rd edition. St Louis (MO): Saunders Elsevier; 2009. p. 487–501.

34. Mayhew J. Neurologic evaluation. In: Large animal neurology. 2nd edition. Oxford (UK): Wiley-Blackwell; 2009. p. 11–46.

35. Furr M, Reed S. Neurologic examination. In: Equine neurology. 1st edition. Oxford (UK): Wiley-Blackwell; 2007. p. 65–76.

36. Johnson AL. How to perform a complete neurologic examination in the field and identify abnormalities. Proc 56th Annu Convent AAEP 2010;56:331–7.

37. Holcombe SJ. Neuromuscular regulation of the larynx and nasopharynx in the horse. Proc Annu Convent AAEP 1998;44:26–9.

38. Baptiste K. Functional anatomy observations of the pharyngeal orifice of the equine guttural pouch (auditory tube diverticulum). Vet J 1997;153:311–9.

39. Holcombe SJ, Derksen FJ, Stick JA, et al. Pathophysiology of dorsal displacement of the soft palate in horses. Equine Vet J 1999;(Suppl 30):45–8.

40. Klebe EA, Holcombe SJ, Rosenstein D, et al. The effect of bilateral glossofaryngeal nerve anesthesia swallowing in horses. Equine Vet J 2005;37:65–9.

41. Holcombe SJ. A review of upper airway anatomy and physiology of the horse. Presented at the Eighth AAEP Annual Resort Symposium; Rome: 2006. p. 19–21.

42. Cheetham J, Pigott JH, Hermanson JW, et al. Role of the hypoglossal nerve in equine nasopharyngeal stability. J Appl Physiol 2009;107:471–7.

43. Janicek JC, Ketzner KM. Airflow mechanics, Upper respiratory diagnostics, and performance-limiting pharyngeal disorders. Compend Equine 2008;366–80.

44. Cohen ND. Neurologic evaluation of the equine head and neurologic dysphagia. Vet Clin North Am Equine Pract 1993;9:199–208.

45. Mayhew IG. Horner's syndrome and lesions involving the sympathetic nervous system. Equine Pract 1980;2:44–7.

46. Hahn CN. Horner's syndrome in horses. Equine Vet Educ 2003;15:86–90.

47. Cook WR. The clinical features of guttural pouch mycosis in the horse. Vet Rec 1968;83:336–45.

48. Merriam JG. Guttural pouch fibroma in a mare. J Am Vet Med Assoc 1972;161:487–9.

49. Trigo FJ, Nickels FA. Squamous cell carcinoma of a horse's guttural pouch. Mod Vet Pract 1981;62:456–9.

50. Sweeney CR, Freeman DE, Sweeney RW, et al. Hemorrhage into the guttural pouch (auditory tube diverticulum) associated with rupture of the longus capitis muscle in three horses. J Am Vet Med Assoc 1993;202:1129–31.

51. Cook WR. Observations on the aetiology of epistaxis and cranial nerve paralysis in the horse. Vet Rec 1966;78:396–405.

52. Kuehn DP, Folkings JW, Cutting CB. Relationships between muscle activity and velar position. Cleft Palate J 1982;19:25–35.

53. Holcombe SJ, Derksen FJ, Robinson NE. Electromyographic activity of the *palatinus* and *palatopharyngeus* muscles in exercising horses. Equine Vet J 2007;39:451–5.

54. Barakzai SZ, Hawkes CS. Dorsal displacement of the soft palate and palatal instability. Equine Vet Educ 2010;22:253–64.

55. Morello SL, Ducharme NG, Hackett RP, et al. Activity of selected rostral and caudal hyoid muscles in clinically normal horses during strenuous exercise. Am J Vet Res 2008;69:682–9.

56. Holcombe SJ, Derksen FJ, Stick JA, et al. Effects of bilateral hypoglossal and glossopharyngeal nerve blocks on epiglottic and soft palate position in exercising horses. Am J Vet Res 1997;58:1022–6.

57. Tessier C, Holcombe SJ, Derkesen FJ. Effects of stylopharyngeus muscle dysfunction on the nasopharynx in exercising horses. Equine Vet J 2004;36:318–23.

58. Mayhew IG. Neurology of recurrent laryngeal neuropathy and the thoraco-laryngeal reflex. In: Dixon P, Robinson E, Wade JF, editors. Proceedings of Workshop on Equine Recurrent Laryngeal Neuropathy: Stratford-upon-Avon, UK; 2003. p. 5–8.

59. Pollock PJ. Diagnosis and management of guttural pouch mycosis. Equine Vet J 2007;19:522–7.

60. Lane JG. The management of guttural pouch mycosis. Equine Vet J 1989;21:321–4.

61. Cook WR, Campbell RS, Dawson C. The pathology and aetiology of guttural pouch mycosis in the horse. Vet Rec 1968;83:422–8.
62. Johnson JH, Merriam JG, Attleberger M. A case of guttural pouch mycosis caused by Aspergillus nidulans. Vet Med Small Anim Clin 1973;68:771–4.
63. Knight AP. Dysphagia resulting from unilateral rupture of the rectus capitis ventralis muscles in a horse. J Am Vet Med Assoc 1977;170:735–8.
64. Björklund NE, Palsson G. Guttural pouch mycosis in the horse. A survey of 7 cases and a case report. Nord Vet-Med 1970;22:65–74.
65. Rawlinson RJ, Jones RT. Guttural pouch mycosis in two horses. Aust Vet J 1978;54: 135–8.
66. Dixon PM, Rowlands AC. Atlanto-occipital joint infection association with guttural pouch mycosis in a horse. Equine Vet J 1981;13:260–2.
67. Hilbert BJ, Huxtable CR, Brighton AJ. Erosion of the internal carotid artery and cranial nerve damage caused by guttural pouch mycosis in a horse. Aust Vet J 1981;57: 346–7.
68. Lane JG, Mair TS. Observations on headshaking in the horse. Equine Vet J 1987;19: 331–6.
69. Greet TRC. Outcome of treatment of 35 cases of guttural pouch mycosis. Equine Vet J 1987;19:483–7.
70. Walmsley JP. A case of atlanto-occipital arthropathy following guttural pouch mycosis in a horse. The use of radioisotope bone scanning as an aid to diagnosis. Equine Vet J 1988;20:219–20.
71. Howarth S, Lane JG. Multiple cranial nerve deficits associated with auditory tube (guttural pouch) diverticulitis: three cases. Equine Vet Educ 1990;2:206–9.
72. Kipar A, Frese K. Hypoglossal neuritis with associated lingual hemiplegia secondary to guttural pouch mycosis. Vet Pathol 1993;30:574–6.
73. Dixon PM, McGorum BC, Railton DI, et al. Laryngeal paralysis: a study of 375 cases in a mixed-breed population of horses. Equine Vet J 2001;33:452–8.
74. Cabañes FJ, Monreal L, Majó N, et al. Micosis de lãs bolsas guturales causada por Emericella nidulans em um caballo. Ver Iberoam Micol 2002;19:208–11.
75. Laugier C, Tapprest J, Foucher N, et al. A necropsy survey of neurologic diseases in 4,319 horses examined in Normandy (France) from 1986 to 2006. J Equine Vet Sci 2009;29:561–8.
76. Laus F, Paggi E, Cerquetella M, et al. Guttural pouch mycosis in a donkey (*Equus asinus*): a case report. Vet Med 2010;55:561–5.
77. Modransky PD, Reed SM, Barbee DD. Dysphagia associated with guttural pouch empyema and dorsal displacement of the soft palate. Equine Pract 1982;4:34–8.
78. McCue PM, Freeman DE, Donawick WJ. Guttural pouch tympany: 15 cases (1977–1986). J Am Vet Med Assoc 1989;194:1761–3.
79. Blazyczek I, Hamann H, Deegen E, et al. Retrospective analysis of 50 cases of guttural pouch tympany in foals. Vet Rec 2004;154:261–4.
80. Greene HJ, O'Connor JP. Haemangioma of the guttural pouch of a 16-year-old thoroughbred mare: clinical and pathological findings. Vet Rec 1986;118:445–6.
81. Baptiste KE, Moll HD, Robertson JL. Three horses with neoplasia including growth in the guttural pouch. Can Vet J 1996;37:499–501.
82. Hatziolos BC, Sass B, Albert TF, et al. Ocular changes in a horse with gutturomycosis. J Am Vet Med Assoc 1975;167:51–4.
83. McConnico RS, Blas-Machado U, Cooper VL, et al. Bilateral squamous cell carcinoma of the guttural pouches and the left middle ear in a horse. Equine Vet Educ 2001;13:175–8.

84. Cook W. Disease of the ear, nose and throat of the horse. Part 1: The ear. In: Grunsell O, editor. The veterinary annual. Bristol, UK: John Wright & Sons; 1971. p. 12–43.

85. Rush BR. Vestibular disease. In: Reed S, Bayly WM, Sellon DC, editors. Equine internal medicine. 2nd edition. St Louis (MO): Saunders; 2004. p. 579–88.

86. McLaughlin BG, O'Brien JL. Guttural pouch mycosis and mycotic encephalitis in a horse. Can Vet J 1986;27:109–11.

87. Wagner PC, Miller RA, Gallins AM, et al. Mycotic encephalitis associated with a guttural pouch mycosis. J Equine Med Surg 1978;2:355–9.

88. Bacon Miller C, Wilson DA, Martim DD, et al. Complications of balloon catherization associated with aberrant cerebral arterial anatomy in a horse with guttural pouch mycosis. Vet Surg 1998;27:450–3.

89. Freeman DE, Staller GS, Maxson AD, et al. Unusual carotid artery branching that prevent arterial occlusions with a balloon-tipped catheter in a horse. Vet Surg 1993;22:531–4.

90. Hardy J, Robertson JT, Wilkie DA. Ischemic optic neuropathy and blindness after arterial occlusion for treatment of guttural pouch mycosis in two horses. J Am Vet Med Assoc 1990;196:1631–4.

91. Bell C. Pharyngeal neuromuscular dysfunction associated with bilateral guttural pouch tympany in a foal. Can Vet J 2007;48:192–4.

92. Freeman DE. Complications of surgery for disease of the guttural pouch. Vet Clin Equine 2009;24:485–97.

93. Freeman DE, Ross MW, Donawick WJ. Steal phenomenon proposed as the cause of blindness after arterial occlusion for treatment of guttural pouch mycosis in horses. J Am Vet Med Assoc 1990;197:811–2.

Update on Infectious Diseases Affecting the Equine Nervous System

Amy L. Johnson, DVM

KEYWORDS

- Equine herpes virus (EHV-1) • West Nile virus (WNV)
- Rabies • Lyme neuroborreliosis • *Anaplasma*
- Equine protozoal myeloencephalitis (EPM)
- *Parelaphostrongylus tenuis* • *Halicephalobus*

VIRAL DISEASES

Equine Herpes Virus 1 (EHV-1) Myeloencephalopathy

EHV-1 infection has received a great deal of attention in the last decade due to several high-profile outbreaks,[1,2] state-mandated quarantines, and recognition of a "neuropathogenic" strain. This alpha-herpesvirus is ubiquitous throughout the world, and most horses over the age of 2 years have been exposed. Latent infections involving the trigeminal ganglia and respiratory tract lymph nodes are common, and stressful events may trigger reactivation. Although primarily a respiratory pathogen, responsible for fever, inappetence, and nasal discharge in young horses, EHV-1 is also associated with abortions, neonatal death, and neurologic disease, known as EHV-1 myeloencephalopathy (EHM). Disease is spread via aerosolization of respiratory secretions or direct contact with infected horses or fomites. Virus moves from respiratory epithelial cells to regional lymph nodes to peripheral blood leukocytes, causing a cell-associated viremia. When virus crosses from leukocytes into endothelial cells of the central nervous system (CNS), it causes vasculitis with hemorrhage and thrombosis that result in hypoxia and ischemia in surrounding CNS tissue. Typical clinical signs include fever, paresis and ataxia (usually worse in pelvic limbs than thoracic limbs), urinary bladder paralysis with urine dribbling, and decreased tail and anal tone with fecal retention. Severely affected horses may become recumbent or show evidence of brainstem involvement.

Arguably the most important discovery in the last decade of EHV-1 research was the association of a point mutation in the EHV-1 genome with outbreaks of EHM.[3] This mutation results in variation of a single amino acid of the DNA polymerase, such

The author has nothing to disclose.

Department of Clinical Studies - New Bolton Center, 382 West Street Road, University of Pennsylvania School of Veterinary Medicine, Kennett Square, PA 19348, USA

E-mail address: amyjohn@vet.upenn.edu

Vet Clin Equine 27 (2011) 573–587

doi:10.1016/j.cveq.2011.08.008

0749-0739/11/$ – see front matter

that "non-neuropathogenic" strains have asparagine (N_{752}) and neuropathogenic strains have aspartic acid (D_{752}). The mutation appears to lead to a greater magnitude and longer duration of leukocyte-associated viremia, which has been proposed to increase the likelihood of viral movement into endothelial cells of the CNS and subsequent EHM.[4,5] Despite the strong association between the neuropathogenic strain and neurologic disease, the non-neuropathogenic strain can also cause EHM, with a recent retrospective study documenting the non-neuropathogenic strain in 24% of horses with neurologic disease.[6]

The prevalence of latent and active EHV-1 infections has been studied. In the Thoroughbred broodmare population of central Kentucky, 54% of 132 sampled mares had latent infections, and 18% of latently infected mares were carrying the neuropathogenic strain.[7] In contrast, examination of a population of horses in California revealed that only 15% of 153 equids were latently infected, suggesting that differences in horse populations, geographical origin, and management practices may significantly influence the prevalence of latent infections.[8] Active EHV-1 shedding has been investigated in high-risk groups, revealing a low prevalence (1%) in adult horses transported over long distances.[9] The overall detection rate (shedders plus nonshedders) was 2.6%, similar to the 3.8% reported from horses at show events and sales.[10]

Antemortem diagnosis of EHV-1 infection is performed most easily through real-time polymerase chain reaction (PCR) testing of respiratory secretions and whole blood.[11,12] Current PCR tests are able to differentiate so designated neuropathogenic strains from non-neuropathogenic strains. Initial EHV-1 infection occurs at the respiratory epithelium, and viral shedding typically persists for 10 to 14 days. Subsequently, infection spreads to white blood cells and a leukocyte-associated viremia develops and persists for about 14 days although at a lower level than the nasal shedding.[13] Therefore, appropriate samples for submission include nasal swabs and whole blood. Although testing only nasal swabs is probably sufficient for outbreak control and confirming EHM, maximal sensitivity in diagnosis is achieved by testing both nasal swabs and whole blood. The postexposure temporal profiles of EHV-1 in nasal secretions and leukocytes do not completely overlap, and it is possible for one test to be positive while the other is negative. CSF analysis can be supportive but not diagnostic; changes are consistent with a vasculopathy and typically consist of a normal to mildly increased nucleated cell count with increased total protein (albuminocytologic dissociation with xanthochromia). Serum neutralization titers with paired samples as well as virus isolation have also been used in diagnosis but are less frequently used since the advent of PCR testing. Postmortem diagnosis is obtained with a combination of histology and confirmatory immunohistochemistry or PCR.

As with many viral infections, initial descriptions of treatment for EHM focused on supportive care, with particular attention to hydration, nutrition, and bladder care (catheterization and treatment of cystitis as warranted). Corticosteroids and non-steroidal anti-inflammatory drugs, as well as antithrombotic agents such as aspirin and pentoxifylline, are frequently used but of unknown benefit. More recently, specific antiviral treatments have been investigated. Enteral administration of acyclovir was associated with high variability in serum–acyclovir–time profiles, a low maximum serum concentration, and poor bioavailability (2.8%), suggesting limited therapeutic benefit for oral administration.[14] Despite these findings, repeated use of acyclovir (20 mg/kg po q 8 h or 10 mg/kg po 5 times daily) during an outbreak situation seemingly was associated with improved outcome, although causality could not be determined.[1] Multiple oral dosing of valacyclovir (40 mg/kg q 8 h) has been investigated; measured plasma acyclovir concentrations were considered high enough potentially to result in therapeutic benefit.[15] However, it remains uncertain whether valacyclovir will be beneficial in naturally occurring EHV-1 cases or outbreaks. One experimental infection study showed decreased clinical signs, particularly when therapy (27 mg/kg q 8 h for 2 days and then 18 mg/kg q 12 h for 7–14 days) was initiated prior to infection.[16] On the other hand, another experimental study showed no difference in clinical signs, viral shedding, or viremia between treated (40 mg/kg q 8 h for 5–7 days) and untreated ponies.[15] Novel treatments, such as RNA interference using small interfering RNA (siRNA), have shown promise in experimental models but require further investigation before application to clinical cases.[17] Prognosis for affected horses is highly variable; mildly affected horses have a fair to good chance for a full recovery, whereas recumbent horses usually do not recover.

No commercial vaccines are labeled for the prevention of neurologic disease. Preliminary research suggested that use of a modified-live virus vaccine (Rhinomune; Boehringer Ingelheim Vetmedica, St Joseph, MO, USA) was more protective against EHM than use of an inactivated vaccine.[18] However, this study used a small number of animals and induced only mild signs of neurologic disease. A more recent study compared the modified-live vaccine Rhinomune to the high-antigen-load killed vaccine Pneumabort-K (Pfizer Animal Health, New York, NY, USA) with a pony challenge model.[19] Both vaccines reduced clinical signs of respiratory disease and nasal viral shedding, and the killed vaccine reduced the number of days of viremia. Despite the use of an optimized vaccination regime, neither vaccine prevented viremia, which may lead to EHM.

When EHV-1 infection is suspected, particularly if one or more horses are showing neurologic disease, immediate steps to prevent spread of infection are warranted.[13] In many, if not all, states, the neurologic form of EHV-1 is a reportable disease, and the state veterinarian should be informed of any potential cases. Early diagnosis of infection is imperative; practitioners should identify laboratories that will perform real-time PCR testing as expeditiously as possible. Affected horses should be isolated, the facility quarantined, and biosecurity protocols instituted. Temperatures should be monitored twice daily and febrile horses should be assumed infected and separated accordingly. Recent outbreaks have shown that even extensive barrier precautions are ineffective in preventing spread of infection when EHM cases are housed in the same building as other horses, and therefore an isolation facility should be used. In general, 21- to 28-day quarantine periods are elected. Alternatively, shorter 14-day quarantine periods can be used if followed by testing of all horses with quantitative real-time PCR analysis for 2 to 4 consecutive days before releasing the quarantine.[2]

West Nile Virus Infection

Encephalomyelitis due to West Nile virus, a flavivirus transmitted by mosquitoes, was first documented in the United States in New York in 1999 and since that time has been seen across the country.[20] Despite the availability of highly protective vaccines as well as natural immunity that has developed since its appearance in the United States, equine cases are still diagnosed every year. The most recent summary from the Centers for Disease Control and Prevention documented 275 reported equine cases in 2009.[21] Equine infections are often subclinical, causing seroconversion in the absence of clinical signs, but they may produce a spectrum of clinical disease ranging from transient neurologic deficits to fulminating fatal encephalitis.[22] Reported clinical signs in horses include fever, paraparesis or tetraparesis and ataxia that may be symmetric or asymmetric, recumbency, and evidence of intracranial disease including vestibular or cerebellar ataxia and behavioral changes.[22] Although by no means pathognomonic for infection, affected horses frequently show muscle fasciculations and tremors.

Antemortem diagnosis of West Nile virus infection in horses currently starts with identification of compatible neurologic signs in a horse that has been in a location in which West Nile virus activity and mosquitoes have been documented. In seasonal climates, cases tend to occur in the mid to late summer and early fall, when mosquito activity peaks. In warmer climates, cases may appear year-round. Analysis of a large outbreak involving 1698 cases in Texas during 2002 revealed the most common clinical signs to be ataxia (69%), abnormal gait (52%), muscle fasciculations (49%), depression (32%), and recumbency (28%).[23] Since clinical signs are not specific for infection, laboratory confirmation is necessary. Antemortem diagnosis is most commonly made by measuring serum immunoglobulin M (IgM) titer using a capture enzyme-linked immunosorbent assay (ELISA). This test has been reported to have a sensitivity of 92% and specificity of 99%.[24] The utility of testing cerebrospinal fluid (CSF) rather than serum with the IgM capture ELISA has been investigated; 100% agreement between CSF and serum testing was seen, with no clear advantage to testing CSF.[25] Postmortem diagnosis most commonly uses histology of the CNS as well as PCR testing or immunohistochemistry.

Treatment of West Nile virus infection in horses consists primarily of supportive care. No antiviral therapies with documented efficacy against this virus are currently available. However, recent studies using both animal models and naturally occurring human patients have documented clinical improvement in neurologic signs when intravenous immune globulin containing specific antibodies against West Nile virus was administered postinfection.[26] The immune globulin appeared to be beneficial even when administered 3 to 5 days postinfection. The efficacy in animal models appears to be dose dependent; an ideal dose for human patients has not yet been established. Hyperimmune West Nile virus equine plasma is commercially available but not licensed by the U.S. Department of Agriculture. Efficacy studies in naturally occurring equine infections have not been performed.

Prognosis for infected horses is variable, with the most important contributing factors appearing to be severity of disease and vaccination status. A retrospective study examining 484 affected horses in Nebraska and Colorado documented a mortality rate of 28%, with the majority of nonsurviving cases (76%) having been euthanized.[27] Recumbent animals that were unable to rise were 78 times as likely to die, and unvaccinated animals were twice as likely to die as were animals vaccinated at least once. Likewise, the aforementioned retrospective study in Texas (1698 cases) reported a mortality rate of 33%, with the majority of nonsurviving cases (71%) having been euthanized.[23] Recumbency was a strong predictor of death, and vaccination (even when inappropriately timed with regard to disease exposure) was protective.

Prevention of West Nile virus infection is centered on appropriate vaccination, as well as environmental control of mosquito populations. Three vaccines have been licensed: an inactivated whole virus vaccine with adjuvant, a recombinant canary pox vector vaccine, and a modified live chimera vaccine expressed in a flavivirus vector. The first two vaccines are labeled for protection against viremia, whereas the chimera vaccine is labeled for prevention of disease. At the time of publication the chimera vaccine was not commercially available; in April 2010, it was recalled by the manufacturer due to increased incidence of anaphylaxis and other adverse effects (http://www.prevenile.com/). Complete vaccination guidelines are provided by the American Association of Equine Practitioners (http://www.aaep.org/wnv.htm).

Eastern, Western, and Venezuelan Equine Encephalomyelitis

There is limited new information regarding these mosquito-borne viral encephalitides. However, practitioners should realize that these diseases still occur in the equine population despite very effective vaccines. In particular, eastern equine encephalitis (EEE) has been reported more frequently in several areas in the last few years, perhaps in part due to the depressed economy and decline in vaccination but also due to favorable environmental conditions. In 2008, EEE was diagnosed in 19 horses in Quebec[28]; in 2009, 15 fatal equine cases of EEE were identified in Maine[29]; and in 2010, Michigan had an unusually high prevalence of EEE (at least 45 confirmed equine cases).[30] Antemortem diagnosis can be attempted with serology, generally using IgM capture ELISAs.[31,32] Specific, effective treatments have not been described. Prognosis is poor, with a high mortality rate.

Rabies

Infection with rabies virus, a rhabdovirus in the genus *Lyssavirus*, has severe consequences for both equine patients, in which disease is almost invariably fatal, and for in-contact people and animals. During 2009, 41 horses were diagnosed with rabies in the United States, as well as 4 human rabies cases.[33] Although the likelihood of a person developing rabies through contact with a rabid horse appears to be very low, the possibility exists as the virus is known to be present in the salivary glands of affected horses.[34] Recently, a veterinarian died from rabies after handling rabid herbivores (cattle and goats).[35] Therefore, suspect cases should be handled with appropriate caution and personal protective equipment, particularly gloves.

Veterinarians should always consider rabies as a possible differential diagnosis when faced with a neurologic horse, particularly one with an unknown or inadequate vaccination history. Signs of rabies are inconsistent and often vague in horses; early cases may show only lameness or colic. Clinical signs of experimentally induced rabies were described in a group of 21 horses and included muzzle tremors, pharyngeal spasm or paresis, ataxia, paresis, lethargy, and somnolence.[36] In the experimental model, average incubation period was 12 days and average morbidity was 5.5 days. Classically, clinical rabies has been divided into furious, dumb, and paralytic forms; 43% of the experimentally infected horses displayed the furious form and none showed the paralytic form, although this form has been described in a naturally occurring case.[37] The largest retrospective case series examined 21 cases of rabies in horses and found a mean survival time after onset of clinical signs of 4.5 days.[38] Initial clinical signs included paraparesis and ataxia (43% cases), lameness (24%), recumbency (14%), pharyngeal paralysis (10%), and colic (10%). Over the course of hospitalization all horses became recumbent (100%) and some became hyperesthetic (81%), lost tail and anal sphincter tone (57%), became febrile (52%), and displayed paraparesis and ataxia (52%). CSF cytology may be normal or abnormal; abnormal samples usually display a mild lymphocytic pleocytosis.

Definitive diagnosis of rabies can only be achieved postmortem. The routine test is the direct fluorescent antibody test on brain specimens. All horses that die or are euthanized after a short (<3-week) course of unexplained progressive neurologic disease should be tested for rabies.

Prevention of rabies is accomplished through adequate vaccination. Three inactivated vaccines are licensed for rabies prophylaxis in horses. Veterinarians are frequently queried regarding the measurement of serum antibody titers as a surrogate marker of protection in place of revaccination. There are insufficient data available to assess the protective value of any given titer, and this author adamantly discourages the practice of recommending titers rather than revaccination. If an unvaccinated horse is exposed to rabies, veterinarians should follow state public health guidelines. Although not universally endorsed, a postexposure rabies prophylaxis protocol, developed and mandated in Texas, has proved to be effective. Over the time period 2000–2009, 72 horses received postexposure prophylaxis and none subsequently developed rabies.[39] This protocol involves immediate vaccination followed by a 90-day isolation period with booster vaccinations during the third and eighth weeks of isolation.

BACTERIAL DISEASES
Anaplasma phagocytophilum Infection (Equine Granulocytic Ehrlichiosis)

Equine granulocytic ehrlichiosis was first reported in the late 1960s in northern California.[40] The causative agent, a coccobacillary gram-negative rickettsial organism with a tropism for neutrophils, was initially named *Ehrlichia equi* but subsequently reclassified as *Anaplasma phagocytophilum*. Infection with *A. phagocytophilum* is transmitted via *Ixodes* spp. ticks and most commonly causes fever, lethargy, inappetence or anorexia, limb edema, icterus, and sometimes petechial hemorrhages. Clinicopathologic changes may include mild anemia, moderate to severe thrombocytopenia, leucopenia, lymphopenia, hyperbilirubinemia, and intracytoplasmic inclusions in neutrophils. Rarely, infection leads to neurologic signs. One horse reportedly became recumbent associated with anaplasmosis; the horse quickly became ambulatory following appropriate treatment (intravenous oxytetracycline).[41] Additionally, a single case of rhabdomyolysis associated with anaplasmosis has been reported. The horse in that report was mildly obtunded with firm, painful musculature and a stiff gait; muscle biopsy results were consistent with myodegeneration and suggestive of oxidative stress.[42]

Based on these case reports, infection with *A. phagocytophilum* should be considered in horses with a stiff gait (ie, with signs of neuromuscular disease) and in ataxic or recumbent horses presenting with fever, particularly if a history of tick exposure and/or hematologic changes consistent with anaplasmosis are present. The presence of intracytoplasmic inclusions in neutrophils on a blood or buffy coat smear provides strong supporting evidence for infection. The most definitive test is PCR on whole blood. Serology may also be helpful, although positive results only indicate exposure and not necessarily active infection. A significant (4-fold or greater) rise in antibody titer between paired blood samples confirms active infection.[40]

In general, clinical improvement is rapidly apparent with appropriate treatment. Oxytetracycline at 7 mg/kg IV once daily for 5 to 7 days is usually effective. Most horses defervesce within 12 to 36 hours of treatment initiation; this response aids in diagnosis. Rarely, horses may relapse after apparently successful treatment, usually when treated for less than 7 days.[43] Untreated horses generally recover spontaneously in terms of clinical signs but may have persistent infections for at least 129 days.[44] It is unclear whether persistent infection occurs in horses treated for at least 7 days.

Borrelia burgdorferi

Infection with *B. burgdorferi*, the causative agent of Lyme disease, is increasingly recognized in horses and ponies in North America. However, diagnosis of clinical disease is challenging because of its variable clinical manifestations as well as serologic test limitations.[45] In all likelihood, many horses are infected with minimal or no clinical signs. Historically, clinical signs attributed to *B. burgdorferi* infection include chronic weight loss, sporadic lameness, stiffness, arthritis, swollen joints, muscle tenderness, hepatitis, laminitis, fever, abortion, uveitis, and encephalitis.[46-48] More recently, several reports describing neuroborreliosis in horses have been published. In the first, an adult Thoroughbred in the United Kingdom showed lethargy, anorexia, pyrexia, ataxia, hyperesthesia, uveitis, and polysynovitis that, despite oxytetracycline treatment, progressed to stupor, recumbency, and dangerous behavior necessitating euthanasia. Necropsy revealed meningoencephalitis with the presence of *Borrelia* confirmed via PCR.[49] In the United States, an adult Thoroughbred was reported to show signs of depression, neck stiffness, and poor performance.[50] CSF analysis revealed a neutrophilic pleocytosis with increased total protein, and Western blot analysis of serum samples obtained 3 days apart revealed conversion from equivocal to low/moderate positive results, consistent with active *B. burgdorferi* infection. Additionally, PCR assay of CSF for *B. burgdorferi* yielded positive results. The gelding initially appeared to respond to treatment with doxycycline and phenylbutazone. However, 60 days after treatment discontinuation, the horse had a recurrence of neurologic signs, including neck stiffness, ataxia, tremors, and unilateral vestibular disease, as well as menace response deficits and periods of abnormal mental status and behavior. These signs rapidly progressed, necessitating euthanasia. Necropsy results revealed lymphohistiocytic leptomeningitis and vasculitis as well as lymphocytic cranial neuritis and peripheral radiculoneuritis.

In the most recent report, two horses with progressive neurologic disease were diagnosed with neuroborreliosis.[51] One horse showed neck and back pain, lumbar hyperesthesia, lethargy, inappetence, weight loss, and uveitis that eventually progressed to ataxia, paresis, facial paralysis, abnormal behavior, and recumbency prior to euthanasia. The other horse showed waxing and waning muscle atrophy, gait deficits, and hyperesthesia that progressed to facial nerve deficits, ataxia, and behavior changes prior to euthanasia. Necropsy results were consistent with meningoencephalitis and radiculoneuritis with varying degrees of necrosis and fibrosis. Borreliosis was confirmed via direct observation of spirochetes, PCR, and immunohistochemistry.

Although neuroborreliosis has been infrequently reported, the prevalence of *Borrelia* exposure in certain areas of the United States suggests that neuroborreliosis should more frequently be considered in the differential diagnosis for horses with neurologic disease, particularly if signs consistent with meningitis, polyradiculoneuritis, or polyneuropathy are observed (neck or back pain, hyperesthesia, muscle atrophy, sensory deficits, cranial nerve deficits). Additional signs that may point toward *Borrelia* include uveitis and polysynovitis. Antemortem diagnosis has most commonly been obtained by serologic testing, frequently via kinetic ELISA and Western blot, but more sophisticated immunologic assays are being introduced for dogs and may soon be validated for horses.[52]

The paucity of reported cases, all of which were euthanized on the basis of progressive clinical disease, does not allow any conclusions regarding treatment of neuroborreliosis. In fact, very little information is available regarding the efficacy of treatment for extraneural involvement. In experimentally infected ponies, oxytetracycline was more effective than ceftiofur or doxycycline at eliminating persistent infection.[53] However, in one of the reported cases,[49] as well as in the author's experience, oxytetracycline (5–10 mg/kg IV q 24 h) is not always successful in cases of neuroborreliosis. Doxycycline (10 mg/kg po q 12 h) may lead to reduction in clinical signs, although relapses are possible once treatment is discontinued.[50] Minocycline (4 mg/kg po q 12 h) shows excellent CNS penetration and may be the most appropriate choice but has not yet been evaluated in clinical cases.[54]

PROTOZOAL DISEASES
Equine Protozoal Myeloencephalitis

Equine protozoal myeloencephalitis (EPM) is one of the most frequently diagnosed neurologic conditions in North America. This disease is most often caused by CNS infection with *Sarcocystis neurona*, although infection with other protozoal species, including *Neospora hughesi*, has also been reported.[55] Horses are infected with *S. neurona* through the consumption of food or water contaminated with opossum feces containing sporocysts. *S. neurona* merozoites may affect any part of the CNS, causing highly variable clinical signs that may manifest insidiously or suddenly and subsequently progress slowly or rapidly. EPM infection is a great mimicker and can rarely be discounted based on clinical signs, although infected horses are typically not in pain or febrile unless comorbidities exist. Many horses show general proprioceptive (spinal) ataxia that is often asymmetric as well as evidence of lower motor neuron involvement, such as lameness or muscle atrophy. Brainstem involvement may manifest as cranial nerve deficits; in this author's experience, dysphagia is a relatively common sign of EPM. A recent retrospective study from the author's veterinary hospital revealed that more referral cases of EPM showed brainstem involvement than any other neuroanatomic location.[56] However, this finding likely does not reflect many ambulatory veterinarians' experience with the disease.

Despite decades of research, EPM remains a diagnostic challenge. Definitive diagnosis requires postmortem confirmation of *S. neurona* infection by microscopic identification, immunohistochemistry, culture, or PCR.[57] Therefore, antemortem diagnosis is always presumptive and considered most accurate if three criteria are fulfilled: compatible clinical signs referable to the CNS, exclusion of other likely diseases, and confirmation of exposure to *S. neurona* by immunologic testing. In areas where *S. neurona* and opossums are common, there is extensive equine exposure to the protozoa, and seroconversion is common. It is extremely important not to base an EPM diagnosis solely on seroconversion, as many horses falsely will be considered positive.

There are several immunologic tests currently in use for EPM diagnosis. All commonly used tests are based on the presence of antibodies in serum or CSF; different tests identify different antibodies. As aforementioned, exposure to the parasite in the absence of CNS infection confounds test interpretation. Even if CSF is analyzed, results may be affected by blood contamination or natural diffusion of antibodies from blood into CSF. The Western blot, a semiquantitative test for antibodies against merozoite lysate, is the oldest and most well-established test. Although the sensitivity of the Western blot is high (about 80%–90%), the specificity is low (about 40%), and minimal blood contamination of CSF may lead to false-positive results.[58,59] The indirect fluorescent antibody test (IFAT), a quantitative test for antibodies against whole merozoites,[60] and the surface antigen 1 (SAG-1) ELISA, a quantitative test based on an immunodominant surface antigen of *S. neurona*,[61] were evaluated recently using naturally occurring cases.[56] Results indicated that the sensitivity of the IFAT (94%) was much higher than that of the SAG-1 ELISA (13%) and that the low sensitivity of the SAG-1 ELISA severely limited its usefulness in the tested patient population. The specificity of the IFAT was also high (85%–90%) in this study. Other work demonstrated that the IFAT, when performed on CSF, is more resilient to blood contamination than the Western blot, with no false-positive results at contamination levels as high as 10,000 red blood cells/μL CSF.[62]

Recent research in parasite biology has elucidated the reason for the poor performance of the SAG-1 ELISA as well as directed new diagnostic efforts.

S. neurona expresses multiple surface antigens (SnSAGs) that serve as virulence factors for the parasite but are immunogenic to the host. SnSAG1 expression is variable, with protozoa expressing either SnSAG1 or SnSAG5 or SnSAG6.[63,64] Logically, horses infected with *S. neurona* strains that do not express SnSAG1 will not produce antibodies that are detectable with the SAG-1 ELISA. SnSAGs 2, 3, and 4 appear to be well-conserved among strains and the most recently marketed EPM tests use monovalent and polyvalent ELISAs to detect antibodies against these three antigens.[65,66] A combination of two assays (rSnSAG2 ELISA and chimeric rSnSAG4/3 ELISA) has been evaluated in a field study using 131 clinical neurologic cases.[67] In this study, a serum-to-CSF ratio was more informative than endpoint CSF titers, with 89% accuracy. Endpoint serum titers were not predictive for a diagnosis of EPM. Although documentation of antibody production remains a surrogate marker of infection, available evidence suggests that measuring specific antibodies in both serum and CSF to allow calculation of a ratio is the most accurate means of diagnosis. In general, antibodies are partitioned between blood and CSF at a relatively constant ratio (100:1), based on the restriction coefficient of the blood-brain barrier. Infection of the CNS leads to intrathecal antibody production and a decrease in this ratio, which is useful in EPM diagnosis.[68]

Four treatments have been approved by the U.S. Food and Drug Administration (FDA) for EPM: a combination of sulfadiazine and pyrimethamine, ponazuril, nitazoxanide, and diclazuril. Efficacy appears similar across treatments but side effects vary. Clinical trials directly comparing the medications and different protocols are sorely needed.

Sulfadiazine at 20 mg/kg and pyrimethamine at 1 mg/kg daily for a minimum of 90 days is the approved combination treatment. When this formulation is commercially unavailable, some practitioners use an extralabel combination of trimethoprim-sulfa tablets (20–30 mg/kg, q 12–24 h po) with pyrimethamine tablets (1 mg/kg q 24 h po). Each of these three drugs (trimethoprim, sulfadiazine, and pyrimethamine) inhibits an enzyme in the folic acid pathway, thereby inhibiting thymidine synthesis. A field study performed during the approval process resulted in successful outcomes in 61.5% of horses, with bone marrow suppression (anemia, leukopenia, neutropenia, and/or thrombocytopenia) as the most common adverse effect.[69] Additional reported side effects may include gastrointestinal side effects (anorexia, depression, glossitis, or diarrhea) and reproductive problems (abortions, changes in copulation or ejaculation, and congenital defects).[70–73]

Ponazuril paste, a triazinetrione antiprotozoal drug, is labeled at 5 mg/kg po daily for 28 days. A field study performed during the approval process described a 60% success rate at the labeled dose.[74] No adverse effects were noted. Anecdotally, ponazuril is used frequently in extralabel dosing regimens, often at significantly higher dosages or for a longer duration. Recent research has indicated that the addition of DMSO to ponazuril (in the form of toltrazuril sulfone powder derived from Baycox) will increase the oral bioavailability threefold and that using a loading dose (5–7 times the maintenance dose) should dramatically decrease the time to reach steady-state levels in CSF (from 10–12 days to 1 day).[75]

Nitazoxanide paste, a 5-nitrothiazole antiparasitic drug, is no longer commercially available. Two field studies for efficacy and safety were performed.[76] The first field study was performed with similar criteria to the field studies for sulfadiazine/pyrimethamine and ponazuril, with similar results, as 57% of treated horses were considered successes. In the second, less-stringent study, 81% of horses were considered treatment successes. Nitazoxanide reportedly has the highest rate of side effects, predominantly gastrointestinal, and the label bears the warning, "Administration of nitazoxanide can disrupt the normal microbial flora of the gastrointestinal tract leading to enterocolitis. Deaths due to enterocolitis have been observed while administering the recommended dose in field studies."

Finally, diclazuril, a triazinetrione antiprotozoal agent similar to ponazuril, has recently been marketed. A field study was performed during the approval process using diclazuril pellets at 1 mg/kg daily for 28 days.[77] Efficacy was similar to the other products with 67% of horses being considered treatment successes, and no important adverse reactions were reported.

PARASITIC DISEASES
Parelaphostrongylus tenuis

P. tenuis is most commonly known as the "meningeal worm" of small ruminants and camelids. White-tailed deer are the definitive hosts of this nematode, which has a complicated life-cycle involving extensive migration through the gastrointestinal tract, CNS, and respiratory tract of the deer as well as migration through gastropod intermediate hosts (snails and slugs). Aberrant hosts show signs of CNS disease when larvae migrate through the spinal cord and/or brain. Horses appear relatively resilient to infection; however, 11 equids with presumptive or confirmed parelaphostrongylosis have been reported.[78–81] Eighty-two percent (9 of 11) of these cases displayed acquired scoliosis due to dorsal gray matter segmental myelitis, while one showed spastic tetraparesis and ataxia consistent with a cervical myelopathy and one had an intraocular infection. The pathogenesis of the acquired scoliosis appears to be neuromuscular in origin; unilateral destruction of the dorsal gray column leads to loss of sensory afferent information on the affected side. Normal muscle tone requires sensory information; without it, the muscles become abnormally flaccid. Subsequent imbalance in cervical muscle tone (flaccid on affected side, normal muscle tone on unaffected side) causes curvature of the neck toward the normal side.

In all reported cases, diagnosis has been presumptive or obtained postmortem. A presumptive diagnosis can be made if the horse shows an acute onset of cervical scoliosis, generally with minimal ataxia and paresis, and other possible etiologies such as EPM and vertebral trauma/malformation are excluded through appropriate immunologic testing, and imaging. As equine *P. tenuis* infection tends to cause segmental unilateral dorsal gray column myelitis, affected horses generally display reduced sensation over the affected side (which is the convex side of the scoliotic curve) and normal sensation over the unaffected side (which is the concave side of the scoliotic curve). CSF analysis may be relatively normal or show mixed pleocytosis. Evaluation of affected spinal cord with magnetic resonance imaging could be very useful in diagnosis but has not yet been described. Definitive diagnosis requires parasite confirmation through visualization of specific parasitic features on histology or molecular confirmation, such as with PCR.[79,82]

Although treatment has been attempted with anthelmintics and anti-inflammatory drugs, successful resolution of infection has not been documented. Based on the severity of necrosis associated with many of the lesions on postmortem exam, complete recovery seems unlikely. However, even horses with severe cervical scoliosis appear comfortable and generally have only mild signs of tetra-ataxia and paresis, so prolonged survival is possible (author, personal experience).

Halicephalobus gingivalis

Infection with the saprophytic nematode *H. gingivalis* (previously *H. deletrix, Micronema deletrix*) is rare but has been reported in horses worldwide. This free-living nematode is suspected to gain entry into the horse via mucosal breaks in the oral cavity. Predilection sites for migration are the kidneys, mandibular region, and CNS. Reported clinical signs include facial swelling, uveitis, lameness, orchitis, renal disease, posthitis, and a variety of CNS deficits.[83] Most reported cases have shown signs referable to brain involvement, although one case demonstrated signs compatible with cauda equina neuritis.[84] Diagnosis of CNS involvement has typically been made at postmortem examination, but advanced imaging techniques such as magnetic resonance imaging potentially could increase suspicion of parasite migration. If horses have extraneural signs (mandibular swelling, renal involvement), biopsy could confirm *Halicephalobus*, and confirmation should raise concerns about impending CNS involvement. Although successful treatment with anthelmintics and/or surgical removal has been reported for horses with extraneural involvement, there are no reports of recovery in horses with CNS involvement.[83]

REFERENCES

1. Henninger RW, Reed SM, Saville WJ, et al. Outbreak of neurologic disease caused by equine herpesvirus-1 at a university equestrian center. J Vet Intern Med 2007;21:157–65.
2. Goehring LS, Landolt GA, Morley PS. Detection and management of an outbreak of equine herpesvirus type 1 infection and associated neurological disease in a veterinary teaching hospital. J Vet Intern Med 2010;24:1176–83.
3. Nugent J, Birch-Machin I, Smith KC, et al. Analysis of equid herpesvirus 1 strain variation reveals a point mutation of the DNA polymerase strongly associated with neuropathogenic versus nonneuropathogenic disease outbreaks. J Virol 2006;80: 4047–60.
4. Allen GP, Breathnach CC. Quantification by real-time PCR of the magnitude and duration of leucocyte-associated viraemia in horses infected with neuropathogenic vs. non-neuropathogenic strains of EHV-1. Equine Vet J 2006;38:252–7.
5. Goodman LB, Loregian A, Perkins GA, et al. A point mutation in a herpesvirus polymerase determines neuropathogenicity. PLoS Pathog 2007;3:e160.
6. Perkins GA, Goodman LB, Tsujimura K, et al. Investigation of the prevalence of neurologic equine herpes virus type 1 (EHV-1) in a 23-year retrospective analysis (1984–2007). Vet Microbiol 2009;139:375–8.
7. Allen GP, Bolin DC, Bryant U, et al. Prevalence of latent, neuropathogenic equine herpesvirus-1 in the Thoroughbred broodmare population of central Kentucky. Equine Vet J 2008;40:105–10.
8. Pusterla N, Mapes S, Wilson WD. Prevalence of equine herpesvirus type 1 in trigeminal ganglia and submandibular lymph nodes of equids examined postmortem. Vet Rec 2010;167:376–9.
9. Pusterla N, Mapes S, Madigan JE, et al. Prevalence of EHV-1 in adult horses transported over long distances. Vet Rec 2009;165:473–5.
10. Yactor J, Lunn KF, Traub-Dargatz JL. Detection of nasal shedding of EHV-1 and 4 at equine show events and sales by multiplex real-time PCR. Proceedings of the 52nd Annual Convention of the American Association of Equine Practitioners, San Antonio, Texas, 2006;223–7.
11. Hussey SB, Clark R, Lunn KF, et al. Detection and quantification of equine herpesvirus-1 viremia and nasal-shedding by real-time polymerase chain reaction. J Vet Diagn Invest 2006;18:335–42.
12. Allen GP. Development of a real-time polymerase chain reaction assay for rapid diagnosis of neuropathogenic strains of equine herpesvirus-1. J Vet Diagn Invest 2007;19:69–72.

13. Lunn DP, Davis-Poynter N, Flaminio MJBF, et al. Equine herpesvirus-1 consensus statement. J Vet Intern Med 2009;23:450–61.
14. Bentz BG, Maxwell LK, Erkert RS, et al. Pharmacokinetics of acyclovir after single intravenous and oral administration to adult horses. J Vet Intern Med 2006;20: 589–94.
15. Garre B, Gryspeerdt A, Croubels S, et al. Evaluation of orally administered valacyclovir in experimentally EHV1-infected ponies. Vet Microbiol 2009;135:214–21.
16. Maxwell LK, Bentz BG, Gilliam LL, et al. Efficacy of valacyclovir against clinical disease after EHV-1 challenge in aged mares. Proceedings of the 54th Annual Convention of the American Association of Equine Practitioners, 2008.
17. Brosnahan MM, Damiani A, van de Walle G, et al. The effect of siRNA treatment on experimental equine herpesvirus type 1 (EHV-1) infection in horses. Virus Res 2010; 147:176–81.
18. Goodman LB, Wagner B, Flaminio MJ, et al. Comparison of the efficacy of inactivated combination and modified-live virus vaccines against challenge infection with neuro-pathogenic equine herpesvirus type 1 (EHV-1). Vaccine 2006;24:3636–45.
19. Goehring LS, Wagner B, Bigbie R, et al. Control of EHV-1 viremia and nasal shedding by commercial vaccines. Vaccine 2010;28:5203–11.
20. Centers for Disease Control and Prevention. Outbreak of West Nile-like viral encepha-litis–New York, 1999. MMWR 1999;48:845–9.
21. Centers for Disease Control and Prevention. West Nile virus activity–United States, 2009. MMWR 2010;59:769–72.
22. Ostlund EN, Andresen JE, Andresen M. West Nile encephalitis. Vet Clin North Am Equine Pract 2000;16:427–41.
23. Ward MP, Schuermann JA, Highfield LD, et al. Characteristics of an outbreak of West Nile virus encephalomyelitis in a previously uninfected population of horses. Vet Microbiol 2006;118:255–9.
24. Long MT, Jeter W, Hernandez J, et al. Diagnostic performance of the equine IgM capture ELISA for serodiagnosis of West Nile virus infection. J Vet Intern Med 2006;20:608–13.
25. Porter MB, Long M, Gosche DG, et al. Immunoglobulin M-capture enzyme-linked immunosorbent assay testing of cerebrospinal fluid and serum from horses exposed to West Nile virus by vaccination or natural infection. J Vet Intern Med 2004;18:866–70.
26. Ben-Nathan D, Samina I, Orr N. High titer human immunoglobulin as a specific therapy against West Nile virus encephalitis. Hum Vaccin 2010;6:279–81.
27. Salazar P, Traub-Dargatz JL, Morley PS, et al. Outcome of equids with clinical signs of West Nile virus infection and factors associated with death. J Am Vet Med Assoc 2004;225:267–74.
28. Chenier S, Cote G, Vanderstock J, et al. An eastern equine encephalomyelitis (EEE) outbreak in Quebec in the fall of 2008. Can Vet J 2010;51:1011–5.
29. Gibney KB, Robinson S, Mutebi JP, et al. Eastern equine encephalitis: an emerging arboviral disease threat, Maine, 2009. Vector Borne Zoonotic Dis. doi:10.1089/vbz.2010.0189.
30. Larkin M. High prevalence of EEE in Michigan. J Am Vet Med Assoc 2010;237:1001.
31. Calisher CH, Mahmud MI, el-Kafrawi AO, et al. Rapid and specific serodiagnosis of western equine encephalitis virus infection in horses. Am J Vet Res 1986;47:1296–9.
32. Sahu SP, Alstad AD, Pedersen DD, et al. Diagnosis of eastern equine encephalomy-elitis virus infection in horses by immunoglobulin M and G capture enzyme-linked immunosorbent assay. J Vet Diagn Invest 1994;6:34–8.

33. Blanton JD, Palmer D, Rupprecht CE. Rabies surveillance in the United States during 2009. J Am Vet Med Assoc 2010;237:646–57.

34. Carrieri ML, Peixoto ZM, Paciencia ML, et al. Laboratory diagnosis of equine rabies and its implications for human postexposure prophylaxis. J Virol Methods 2006;138: 1–9.

35. Brito MG, Chamone TL, Silva FJ, et al. Antemortem diagnosis of human rabies in a veterinarian infected when handling a herbivore in Minas Gerais, Brazil. Rev Inst Med Trop Sao Paulo 2011;53:39–44.

36. Hudson LC, Weinstock D, Jordan T, et al. Clinical presentation of experimentally induced rabies in horses. Zentralbl Veterinarmed B 1996;43:277–85.

37. O'Toole D, Mills K, Ellis J, et al. Poliomyelomalacia and ganglioneuritis in a horse with paralytic rabies. J Vet Diagn Invest 1993;5:94–7.

38. Green SL, Smith LL, Vernau W, et al. Rabies in horses: 21 cases (1970–1990). J Am Vet Med Assoc 1992;200:1133–7.

39. Wilson PJ, Oertli EH, Hunt PR, et al. Evaluation of a postexposure rabies prophylaxis protocol for domestic animals in Texas: 2000-2009. J Am Vet Med Assoc 2010;237: 1395–401.

40. Madigan JE, Pusterla N. Ehrlichial diseases. Vet Clin North Am Equine Pract 2000; 16:487–99.

41. Nolen-Walston RD, D'Oench SM, Hanelt LM, et al. Acute recumbency associated with *Anaplasma phagocytophilum* infection in a horse. J Am Vet Med Assoc 2004; 224:1964–6.

42. Hilton H, Madigan JE, Aleman M. Rhabdomyolysis associated with *Anaplasma phagocytophilum* infection in a horse. J Vet Intern Med 2008;22:1061–4.

43. Madigan JE, Gribble D. Equine ehrlichiosis in northern California: 49 cases (1968–1981). J Am Vet Med Assoc 1987;190:445–8.

44. Franzen P, Aspan A, Egenvall A, et al. Molecular evidence for persistence of *Anaplasma phagocytophilum* in the absence of clinical abnormalities in horses after recovery from acute experimental infection. J Vet Intern Med 2009;23:636–42.

45. Johnson AL, Divers TJ, Chang YF. Validation of an in-clinic enzyme-linked immunosorbent assay kit for diagnosis of *Borrelia burgdorferi* infection in horses. J Vet Diagn Invest 2008;20:321–4.

46. Burgess EC. *Borrelia burgdorferi* infection in Wisconsin horses and cows. Ann NY Acad Sci 1988;539:235–43.

47. Butler CM, Houwers DJ, Jongejan F, et al. *Borrelia burgdorferi* infections with special reference to horses: a review. The Veterinary Quarterly 2005;27:146–56.

48. Magnarelli LA, Anderson JF, Shaw E, et al. Borreliosis in equids in northeastern United States. Am J Vet Res 1988;49:359–62.

49. Hahn CN, Mayhew IG, Whitwell KE, et al. A possible case of Lyme borreliosis in a horse in the UK. Equine Vet J 1996;28:84–8.

50. James FM, Engiles JB, Beech J. Meningitis, cranial neuritis, and radiculoneuritis associated with *Borrelia burgdorferi* infection in a horse. J Am Vet Med Assoc 2010;237:1180–5.

51. Imai DM, Barr BC, Daft B, et al. Lyme neuroborreliosis in 2 horses. Vet Pathol 2011 Apr 1. [Epub ahead of print] doi:10.1177/0300985811398246.

52. Wagner B, Freer H, Rollins A, et al. A fluorescent bead-based multiplex assay for the simultaneous detection of antibodies to *B. burgdorferi* outer surface proteins in canine serum. Vet Immunol Immunopathol 2011;140:190–8.

53. Chang YF, Ku YW, Chang CF, et al. Antibiotic treatment of experimentally *Borrelia burgdorferi*-infected ponies. Vet Microbiol 2005;107:285–94.

54. Schnabel LV, Fortier LA, Papich MG, et al. Pharmacokinetics and distribution of minocycline into the plasma, synovial fluid, cerebral spinal fluid and aqueous humor after oral administration of multiple doses in horses. Poster presentation, ACVS Veterinary Symposium, 2010.

55. Finno CJ, Aleman M, Pusterla N. Equine protozoal myeloencephalitis associated with neosporosis in 3 horses. J Vet Intern Med 2007;21:1405–8.

56. Johnson AL, Burton AJ, Sweeney RW. Utility of 2 immunological tests for antemortem diagnosis of equine protozoal myeloencephalitis (Sarcocystis neurona infection) in naturally occurring cases. J Vet Intern Med 2010;24:1184–9.

57. Furr M, MacKay R, Granstrom D, et al. Clinical diagnosis of equine protozoal myeloencephalitis (EPM). J Vet Intern Med 2002;16:618–21.

58. Daft BM, Barr BC, Gardner IA, et al. Sensitivity and specificity of western blot testing of cerebrospinal fluid and serum for diagnosis of equine protozoal myeloencephalitis in horses with and without neurologic abnormalities. J Am Vet Med Assoc 2002;221: 1007–13.

59. Miller MM, Sweeney CR, Russell GE, et al. Effects of blood contamination of cerebrospinal fluid on Western blot analysis for detection of antibodies against Sarcocystis neurona and on albumin quotient and immunoglobulin G index in horses. J Am Vet Med Assoc 1999;215:67–71.

60. Duarte PC, Daft BM, Conrad PA, et al. Comparison of a serum indirect fluorescent antibody test with two Western blot tests for the diagnosis of equine protozoal myeloencephalitis. J Vet Diagn Invest 2003;15:8–13.

61. Ellison SP, Kennedy T, Brown KK. Development of an ELISA to detect antibodies to rSAG1 in the horse. Int J Appl Res Vet Med 2003;1:318–27.

62. Finno CJ, Packham AE, Wilson WD, et al. Effects of blood contamination of cerebrospinal fluid on results of indirect fluorescent antibody tests for detection of antibodies against Sarcocystis neurona and Neospora hughesi. J Vet Diagn Invest 2007;19: 286–9.

63. Crowdus CA, Marsh AE, Saville WJ, et al. SnSAG5 is an alternative surface antigen of Sarcocystis neurona strains that is mutually exclusive to SnSAG1. Vet Parasitol 2008;158:36–43.

64. Wendte JM, Miller MA, Nandra AK, et al. Limited genetic diversity among Sarcocystis neurona strains infecting southern sea otters precludes distinction between marine and terrestrial isolates. Vet Parasitol 2010;169:37–44.

65. Hoane JS, Morrow JK, Saville WJ, et al. Enzyme-linked immunosorbent assays for detection of equine antibodies specific to Sarcocystis neurona surface antigens. Clin Diagn Lab Immunol 2005;12:1050–6.

66. Yeargan MR, Howe DK. Improved detection of equine antibodies against Sarcocystis neurona using polyvalent ELISAs based on the parasite SnSAG surface antigens. Vet Parasitol 2011;176:16–22.

67. Reed SM, Howe DK, Yeargan MR, et al. New quantitative assays for the differential diagnosis of equine protozoal myeloencephalitis (EPM). EPM Special Interest Group (SIG) at American College of Veterinary Internal Medicine Forum, 2010.

68. Furr M, Howe D, Reed S, et al. Antibody coefficients for the diagnosis of equine protozoal myeloencephalitis. J Vet Intern Med 2011;25:138–42.

69. Animal Health Pharmaceuticals. Freedom of information summary, NADA 141–240. REBALANCE Antiprotozoal Oral Suspension (sulfadiazine and pyrimethamine) "for the treatment of horses with equine protozoal myeloencephalitis (EPM) caused by Sarcocystis neurona." St Joseph (MT): Animal Health Pharmaceuticals; 2004.

70. Fenger CK, Granstrom DE, Langemeier JL, et al. Epizootic of equine protozoal myeloencephalitis on a farm. J Am Vet Med Assoc 1997;210:923–7.

71. Piercy RJ, Hinchcliff KW, Reed SM. Folate deficiency during treatment with orally administered folic acid, sulphadiazine and pyrimethamine in a horse with suspected equine protozoal myeloencephalitis (EPM). Equine Vet J 2002;34:311–6.

72. Bedford SJ, McDonnell SM. Measurements of reproductive function in stallions treated with trimethoprim-sulfamethoxazole and pyrimethamine. J Am Vet Med Assoc 1999;215:1317–9.

73. Toribio RE, Bain FT, Mrad DR, et al. Congenital defects in newborn foals of mares treated for equine protozoal myeloencephalitis during pregnancy. J Am Vet Med Assoc 1998;212:697–701.

74. Furr M, Kennedy T, MacKay R, et al. Efficacy of ponazuril 15% oral paste as a treatment for equine protozoal myeloencephalitis. Vet Ther 2001;2:215–22.

75. Dirikolu L, Karpiesiuk W, Lehner AF, et al. Synthesis and detection of toltrazuril sulfone and its pharmacokinetics in horses following administration in dimethylsulfoxide. J Vet Pharmacol Ther 2009;32:368–78.

76. IDEXX Pharmaceuticals, Inc. Freedom of information summary, NADA 141–178. NAVIGATOR (32% nitazoxanide) Antiprotozoal Oral Paste "for the treatment of horses with equine protozoal myeloencephalitis (EPM) caused by *Sarcocystis neurona*." Greensboro (NC): IDEXX Pharmaceuticals; 2003.

77. Schering-Plough Animal Health Corporation. Freedom of information summary, NADA 141–268. PROTAZIL Anti-protozoal Pellets (1.56% diclazuril) "for the treatment of equine protozoal myeloencephalitis (EPM) caused by Sarcocystis neurona in horses." Langehorne (PA): Schering-Plough Animal Health Corporation; 2007.

78. Van Biervliet J, de Lahunta A, Ennulat D, et al. Acquired cervical scoliosis in six horses associated with dorsal grey column chronic myelitis. Equine Vet J 2004;36:86–92.

79. Tanabe M, Kelly R, de Lahunta A, et al. Verminous encephalitis in a horse produced by nematodes in the family protostrongylidae. Vet Pathol 2007;44:119–22.

80. Johnson AL, de Lahunta A, Divers TJ. Acquired scoliosis in horses: case series and proposed pathogenesis. AAEP Proc 2008;54:192–7.

81. Reinstein SL, Lucio-Forster A, Bowman DD, et al. Surgical extraction of an intraocular infection of *Parelaphostrongylus tenuis* in a horse. J Am Vet Med Assoc 2010;237:196–9.

82. Tanabe M, Gerhold RW, Beckstead RB, et al. Molecular confirmation of *Parelaphostrongylus tenuis* infection in a horse with verminous encephalitis. Vet Pathol 2010;47:759.

83. Ferguson R, van Dreumel T, Keystone JS, et al. Unsuccessful treatment of a horse with mandibular granulomatous osteomyelitis due to *Halicephalobus gingivalis*. Can Vet J 2008;49:1099–103.

84. Johnson JS, Hibler CP, Tillotson KM, et al. Radiculomeningomyelitis due to *Halicephalobus gingivalis* in a horse. Vet Pathol 2001;38:559–61.

Metabolic Causes of Encephalopathy in Horses

Thomas J. Divers, DVM

KEYWORDS

- Metabolic • Encephalopathy • Ammonia • Sodium
- Glucose • Horse

PRIMARY HYPERAMMONEMIA ASSOCIATED WITH INTESTINAL DISEASE

Hyperammonemia secondary to intestinal disease or dysfunction appears to be more common in horses than in other species.[1–5] The reason for the relatively high incidence of this disease in horses is unknown. The exact cause of the disorder is also unknown but is presumed to be a result of excessive ammonia production within the intestinal tract. The hypothesis is that this excessive production and absorption of ammonia would overwhelm normal liver metabolism causing ammonia toxicity and the encephalopathic signs. There is some possibility that intestinal overgrowth of hyperammonia-producing bacteria may be responsible for the disorder although no specific bacteria have been documented to be associated with the condition. Overgrowth of specific hyperammonia-producing bacteria and increases in intestinal pH are known to increase intestinal ammonia production in cattle, although neurologic signs were not reported in the cattle.[6] Most horses with the hyperammonemia encephalopathy exhibit either colic and/or diarrhea during or preceding the neurologic signs.[1–5] This provides circumstantial evidence of intestinal dysfunction or disease being associated with the presumed overgrowth of the hyperammonia-producing bacteria and/or increased absorption of ammonia. A recent epidemiologic investigation of 13 documented cases did not find any breed or gender predisposition to the disease; the average age was 12 years (range 4–24 years).[7] Most cases presented between March and October, and most affected horses had access to pasture but no specific type of pasture, hay, or grain could be found in common to all cases. In cattle, there are more hyperammonia-producing bacteria in forage-fed cattle than in grain-fed cattle, which might be consistent with the evidence that most horses with hyperammonemia are not on a high grain diet.[6] In most reports, only a single horse on the farm is affected, although in one report, 2 horses on a single small farm were affected on the same day.[2] One recent report has also identified 10 foals with intestinal hyperammonemia.[8]

The author has nothing to disclose.
Department of Clinical Sciences, College of Veterinary Medicine, Cornell University, Ithaca, NY 14853, USA
E-mail address: tjd8@cornell.edu

Vet Clin Equine 27 (2011) 589–596
doi:10.1016/j.cveq.2011.08.004
0749-0739/11/$ – see front matter © 2011 Elsevier Inc. All rights reserved.

Clinical Signs

A majority of horses with primary hyperammonemia encephalopathy are initially examined for gastrointestinal upset, either colic, diarrhea, or both. Twelve to 24 hours later, the horses characteristically show encephalopathic signs including blindness with dilated pupils that are weakly responsive to light and/or head pressing and/or exhibit bizarre behavior. Diarrhea and protein-losing enteropathy of 1 to 4 days duration are common following onset or resolution of the encephalopathy.

Pathophysiology, Laboratory Findings, and Diagnosis

The excessive absorption of ammonia overwhelms the normal liver causing increases in both plasma and cerebrospinal fluid (CSF) ammonia concentrations. Ammonia concentrations in these 2 fluids have been similar and between 250 and 650 μmol/L. Excessive ammonia in the brain and CSF cause increases in glutamine concentrations leading to astrocyte damage, cerebral swelling, and, if prolonged, death of cerebral neurons.[9,10]

Glutamine synthesis is the major pathway of ammonia detoxification in the brain and CSF. Cerebral energy deficits and oxidative injury are also thought to be involved in the pathophysiology of the disorder.[9] In humans with hyperammonemia, cerebral edema is a feature of the disease, and although this may also be true in horses, it is not documented. The most common microscopic finding in the brain of horses with the disease is the presence of Alzheimer type II cells, which are enlarged astrocytes with basophilic nuclei.[11]

The laboratory findings are a characteristic triad of marked hyperammonemia, metabolic acidosis, and hyperglycemia.[2] The hyperammonemia is thought to be directly responsible for the L-lactic acidosis and the hyperglycemia.[12,13] Identical findings have been reported in ruminants with urea or ammonia poisoning.[12] Hematocrit is generally increased, most likely because of splenic contraction and dehydration. Ammonia can be measured at veterinary hospitals that have an IDEXX VetTest[7] (IDEXX Laboratories, Portland, ME, USA) chemistry analyzer. Blood samples for ammonia testing need to be separated immediately after collection, with plasma stored on ice, and tested within 2 hours after collection. If the horse needs to be euthanized or has died due to the clinical severity, then aqueous humor should be collected in a heparin tube, placed on ice, and tested within 2 hours.

Treatment

Sedation may be required as the initial treatment in order to control the propulsive walking not responsive to manual restraint. Detomidine (10–20 μg/kg IV) may be needed to sedate the affected horse. A dosage that quiets the horse but does not cause excessive lowering of the head would be ideal since lowering of the head might promote cerebral edema. Phenobarbital (5–10 mg/kg IV) may be required to maintain sedation for a more prolonged period. An intravenous catheter should be placed in the jugular vein following the detomidine and intravenous crystalloids with 40 mEq/L of additional KCl administered to correct intravascular volume deficits and electrolyte abnormalities. One dose of hypertonic saline (2 mL/kg) can be given to correct mild hyponatremia and hypochloremia and rapidly improve intravascular volume; also it may decrease cerebral edema (if present). The horse should receive 20 mg/kg neomycin and/or 0.2 mL/kg lactulose via either oral dose syringe or nasogastric tube. Approximately 50% of affected horses are better within 24 hours and have normal neurologic function in 48 hours. Diarrhea and a decline in plasma protein concentration may persist for a couple of days, which may require continued treatments. Some horses with hyperammonemia become comatose and these cases have a very guarded prognosis. Treatment of self-inflicted trauma and tetanus prophylaxis are often required. The only other hyperammonemia syndromes without anatomic or pathologic abnormalities in the liver are hyperammonemia of Morgan foals, which is assumed to be a genetic urea cycle defect, and occasionally meconium impactions in foals.[14]

HEPATIC ENCEPHALOPATHY

Horses with hepatic encephalopathy caused by liver failure or foals with portosystemic encephalopathy have a similar but more complex neuropathophysiology. The encephalopathy in those cases may be a result of hyperammonemia or a multitude of other gut-derived neurotoxins, endogenous false neurotransmitters, increases in aromatic amino acids, hypoglycemia and blood-brain barrier disruption, and additional proposed mechanisms.[15] Brain lesions with hepatic encephalopathy and portosystemic encephalopathy or even uremic encephalopathy are nearly identical to those of primary hyperammonemia. Treatments used to treat primary hyperammonemia are also used as part of the treatment plan for hepatic encephalopathy and portosystemic encephalopathy. The prognosis for hepatic encephalopathy is variable but generally not as good as with primary hyperammonemia. Portosystemic encephalopathy is rare but does occur in foals.[16]

HYPONATREMIA

Sodium disorders, either hyponatremia or hypernatremia, may cause neurologic disorders in most species including the horse. Hyponatremia is the most common of the 2 in the equine and occurs mostly in foals with urinary tract abnormalities or diarrhea and somewhat less commonly in adult horses with diarrhea or renal failure. Common specific conditions include ureteral dilatation with hydronephrosis in foals or acute tubular nephrosis (often due to nephrotoxic drugs), both of which are presumed to cause a salt-losing nephropathy with continued low-sodium fluid intake. Severe diarrhea of 2 or more days is also a common cause due to electrolyte loss in the feces and consumption of a low-sodium fluid (mare's milk and/or water). These disorders are likely due to sodium loss in the urine and/or feces in the face of dehydration and increase in vasopressin (antidiuretic hormone) causing a relative excessive plasma water in comparison to plasma sodium.[17,18] The extracellular fluid volume can be low, normal, or even high in patients with hyponatremia. It is important to note that vasopressin release can be triggered by several physiologic mechanisms, 2 of which are intravascular volume deficits (hemodynamic) and osmotic stimuli (hypernatremia). In dehydrated and hyponatremic animals, the body will attempt to correct the extracellular volume deficit (via increased ADH-driven water absorption) at the expense of the low serum sodium.[18] Ruptured bladder in foals may also cause a severe hyponatremia due to equilibration of sodium into an expanded extracellular fluid volume; this would be a relative water overload causing the hyponatremia. A relative water overload and marked plasma hyponatremia may also occur in horses or foals with protein-losing enteropathy or nephropathy and clinically apparent edema. Although plasma sodium is low in patients with severe edema, total body sodium may be high due to the expansion of the extracellular fluid volume, and treatment with high-sodium fluids may result in worsening of the edema. Neurologic signs associated with hyponatremia appear to be more common in foals than in adult horses.[19] The primary pathology of severe hyponatremia (often <120 mEq/L) is cerebral edema. The hypo-osmolality of the extracellular fluid results in an influx of water into cells, including neurons, causing cytotoxic or intracellular cerebral edema.[20]

Clinical Signs and Treatments

Clinical signs include depression, blindness, ataxia, head pressing, and seizures.[19,20] These clinical findings in addition to serum sodium of <120 mEq/L are suggestive of hyponatremic encephalopathy. Although not documented in horses, a noncardiogenic pulmonary edema may be a rare finding with hyponatremic encephalopathy in humans.[20] There is controversy regarding the preferred treatment of hyponatremic encephalopathy and, prior to selecting the treatment fluid, consideration should be given to the severity and duration of both the hyponatremia and intravascular volume deficits (dehydration). The preferred treatment in most acute cases of severe hyponatremia with intravascular volume depletion is administration of hypertonic sodium chloride, most often 2% to 3% NaCl, although 7.5% could be used in adult horses with severe acute dehydration and hyponatremia. Hypertonic NaCl will more quickly reestablish intravascular volume than will an isotonic crystalloid. It will also help reduce neuronal cytotoxic edema and improve brain perfusion.[20] The hypertonic saline can be given as a 1- to 2-mL/kg bolus in order to rapidly improve perfusion and urine production and decrease cerebral edema. This should be continued at a slower rate once the sodium is increased 10 to 12 mEq/L but remains <125 mEq/L. In human medicine, use of 3% NaCl (2 mL/kg bolus) is standard treatment for neonatal encephalopathy.[20] I have used a slightly more conservative treatment for foals, especially if the severe hyponatremia is chronic (≥2 days) as rapid correction of chronic hyponatremia carries a higher theoretical risk of demyelination syndrome.[21] I am conservative in the speed of correcting severe hyponatremia in foals, even when acute, because of clinical and experimental evidence that serum sodium increases may be more dramatic in neonatal foals receiving crystalloids than what occurs in human neonates. This difference could be due to higher aldosterone concentrations in sick foals than in critically ill human neonates or adult horses.[22] The greatest concern with rapid or overcorrection of hyponatremia in human neonates is the perceived risk of developing cerebral demyelination (osmotic or central pontine myelinolysis).[22] The risk of this occurring in foals is unknown, but due to the paucity of reports in the literature[19] and experiences, this would appear to relatively low. Neonates with more prolonged periods of severe hyponatremia are believed to be at greatest risk. The classic clinical scenario, although rare in children, would be initial improvement in the hyponatremic encephalopathy followed by a neurologic deterioration 2 to 7 days following correction of the hyponatremia.[20] If dehydration is not accompanying the hyponatremia, as may occur in foals with rupture of the bladder, 0.9% NaCl (with additional glucose to counteract hyperkalemia) should be appropriate.

Although hyponatremic encephalopathy is most common in foals, it may on rare occasions occur in adult horses. Horses with colitis and renal failure occasionally develop hyponatremic encephalopathy demonstrating both cerebral dysfunction and ataxia in association with severe hyponatremia (<115 mEq/L).

HYPERNATREMIC ENCEPHALOPATHY

Hypernatremic encephalopathy is much less common than is hyponatremic encephalopathy in foals. Hypernatremic encephalopathy is caused by a sequence of rapid (within hours) production of amino acids (idiosmoles) in the neurons in an attempt to protect against intracellular dehydration in face of the high extracellular fluid osmolality created by the hypernatremia.[17] Too-rapid correction of the plasma hypernatremia may then result in movement of water into the neurons causing cerebral edema. There is little published information on correcting severe (>170 mEq/L) hypernatremia in foals and horses due to the relative rarity of the conditions but we have extensive experience with this in calves in which the condition is common.[23,24] Correction of the hypernatremia should be slow (<0.5 mEq/L/hr has been commonly recommended as a guideline) and via intravenous administration of a fluid that is slightly hypotonic in comparison to the plasma osmolality.[25] Monitoring of "in and out" fluid volume is also important.

KERNICTERUS

Kernicterus is damage to the brain of infants caused by increased levels of unconjugated bilirubin. The condition appears to be uncommon in foals, being reported only rarely with neonatal isoerythrolysis.[26] Marked increases in unconjugated bilirubin quickly saturate plasma protein receptors and the lipid-soluble free unconjugated bilirubin crosses the blood-brain barrier, enters neurons, and induces necrosis. Other physiologic abnormalities such as anemia and hypoxia or hypoglycemia may increase the bilirubin neurotoxicity. Clinical signs in foals include severe icterus, and seizures often resulting in coma. Laboratory findings often include severe anemia, marked bilirubinemia (>30 mg/dL) with increases in mostly unconjugated but some increase in conjugated bilirubin, also. In foals with severe neonatal isoerythrolysis, the liver may be adversely affected by hypoxia, excessive iron pigment, or cholestasis and liver disease can be significant in foals with this disease. Yellow-golden material can be seen in the brain at necropsy in foals with kernicterus. Treatments for kernicterus are unlikely to be successful but crystalloid fluid therapy and either whole blood or oxyglobin can be given in hopes of maintaining perfusion and oxygen-carrying capacity to all organs, especially the brain. In addition, antioxidants and vitamins such as vitamin C, thiamine, and vitamin E may be administered. Plasma transfusion to increase protein binding or plasma exchange could be attempted but the prognosis is poor.

HYPOGLYCEMIA AND CEREBRAL DYSFUNCTION

Hypoglycemia is a common finding in sick neonatal foals. It is most common in neonatal foals with sepsis and systemic inflammation[27] but may also be seen in foals with neonatal encephalopathy syndrome (hypoxic-ischemic encephalopathy or "dummy foals") or starvation and is expected in the rare case of liver failure in foals. Severe hypoglycemia is rare in equines of other ages, although it may occur with chronic debilitating disorders such as neoplasia or chronic intestinal disorders. In one study, foals with critical illness and blood glucose <50 mg/dL on hospital admission were less likely to survive than were critically ill foals with normal blood glucose concentrations.[27] Although glucose is the primary cerebral fuel source, the metabolic consequences of hypoglycemia on the brain are not well known. With severe hypoglycemia, there may be a compensatory increase in cerebral blood flow, and glutamine, pyruvate, acetate, hydroxygluterate, and lactate may provide alternative sources of energy.[28] The increased arterial flow to the hypoglycemic brain will additionally provide some increased glucose availability, and the brain does not require insulin for glucose uptake. In humans with short-term hypoglycemic episodes, magnetic resonance imaging (MRI) lesions seen are often transient and reversible. With more prolonged hypoglycemia, permanent lesions in the occipital lobe of the cerebral cortex and basal ganglia may occur.[29] MRI evaluation of a large number of foals with hypoglycemia has not been reported, but this imaging modality may be useful in detecting lesions and providing prognostic information in foals with hypoglycemia that do not respond to glucose treatment. The clinical signs of hypoglycemia in foals are mostly those of weakness and depression, although seizures may occur.

Treatment of Hypoglycemia

Foals with severe hypoglycemia (<20 mg/dL) should be treated similarly to what is recommended in children with hypoglycemia, with 2 mL/kg of 10% dextrose.[30] This should be followed with a slower continuous intravenous infusion of a 10% dextrose/polyionic fluid. The rate of this infusion is best determined by frequent glucose monitoring (Alpha TRAK System; Abbott, Abbott Park, IL, USA) in addition to other physiologic parameters (intravascular volume, blood pressure, urine production, etc.). For refractory cases, treatment with hydrocortisone (2 mg/kg IV q 12 h) may be attempted. Do not abruptly stop glucose infusion until an enteral source is available and continued blood glucose monitoring confirms that blood glucose has been stabilized within normal range. Marked overcorrection of hypoglycemia should be avoided as the osmotic effects of glucose can be detrimental, and in critically ill children and foals marked hyperglycemia is known to be associated with a lower prognosis.[31,32] Treatment causing mild hyperglycemia (130–170 mg/dL) is unlikely to be a problem, and this mild to moderate hyperglycemia has even been shown to be safe in patients (humans) with brain injury.[32]

Hypoglycemia may be involved in the progressive neurologic dysfunction in hypoxic ischemia encephalopathy, commonly called neonatal encephalopathy.[33] This disorder appears to be a complex and variable perinatal disorder involving an ischemic, hypoxic, inflammatory, apoptotic, oxidative, and metabolic pathophysiology, making the evaluation of any single treatment difficult to determine.[34] Many treatments are used for equine neonatal encephalopathy including mannitol, dimethylsulfoxide (DMSO), thiamine, vitamin C, corticosteroids, allopurinol, magnesium sulfate, benzodiazepines and/or barbiturates for seizure control, slightly raised head position, and maintenance of normal glucose levels, electrolytes, and blood gases.[34] It is difficult to determine which of the treatments are most effective in foals because there are no controlled studies.[35] I prefer treatment with barbiturates (after immediate control of any seizure with a benzodiazepine), mannitol, correction of any oxygen or perfusion deficits, modest head elevation, and magnesium sulfate. Hypothermia and minocycline are potential therapies used in human neonatology, but to my knowledge, they have not been widely applied to the treatment of foals with neonatal encephalopathy.[34]

HYPOCALCEMIC SEIZURE IN GROWING FOALS

This is a rare and often persistent disorder of young growing foals (most often 2–5 weeks of age).[36] The age of onset, consistent with research in other species, suggests efficacy of intestinal absorption and renal handling of calcium may not be mature in the first weeks of life.[37] It may be that the hypocalcemic foals have primary hypoparathyroidism, chronic magnesium deficiency (which decreases parathyroid hormone function), or, less likely, vitamin D deficiency. Seizure and signs of neuromuscular irritability are the characteristic signs in foals with severe hypocalcemia (ionized calcium of <0.6 mmol/L or total calcium <7 mg/dL). Plasma phosphorus concentration is often increased in affected foals, further supporting hypoparathyroidism and not vitamin D deficiency in the disease process. Serum calcium concentration and clinical signs in foals usually responds to 1 to 2 mL/kg calcium borogluconate mixed in 1 L of 0.9% saline, but relapses are expected and most foals are euthanized after repeated episodes. Treatment with intramuscularly administered vitamin D and oral supplementation with magnesium oxide is recommended. Some cases, especially those associated with diarrhea or idiopathic epilepsy as a presumed precipitating factor, have only one episode of hypocalcemic seizure or tetany.

REFERENCES

1. Mair TX. Ammonia and encephalopathy in the horse. Equine Vet J 1997;29:1–2.
2. Peek SF, Divers TJ, Jackson CJ. Hyperammonaemia associated with encephalopathy and abdominal pain without evidence of liver disease in four mature horses. Equine Vet J 1997;29:70–4.
3. Stickle JE, McKnight CA, Williams KJ, et al. Diarrhea and hyperammonemia in a horse with progressive neurologic signs. Vet Clin Pathol 2006;35:250–3.
4. Sharkey LC, DeWitt S, Stockman C. Neurologic signs and hyperammonemia in a horse with colic. Vet Clin Pathol 2006;35:254–8.
5. Gilliam LL, Holbrook TC, Dechant JE, et al. Postmortem diagnosis of idiopathic hyperammonemia in a horse. Vet Clin Pathol 2007;36:196–9.
6. Rychlik JL, Russell JB. Mathematical estimations of hyper-ammonia producing ruminal bacteria and evidence for bacterial antagonism that decreases ruminal ammonia production(1). FEMS Microbiol Ecol 2000;32:121–8.
7. Mittle LD, Hunyadi LM, Divers TJ. Idiopathic hyperammonemia in adult horses [abstract]. Tenth International Equine Colic Research Symposium, Indianapolis, July 2011.
8. Dunkel B, Chaney KP, Dallap-Schaer BL, et al. Putative intestinal hyperammonaemia in horses: 36 cases. Equine Vet J 2011;43:133–40.
9. Auron A, Brophy PD. Hyperammonemia in review: pathophysiology, diagnosis, and treatment. Pediatr Nephrol 2011;26. [Epub ahead of print].
10. Albrecht J, Zielin'ska M, Norenberg MD. Glutamine as a mediator of ammonia neurotoxicity: a critical appraisal. Biochem Pharmacol 2010;80:1303–8.
11. Hasel KM, Summers BA, De Lahunta A. Encephalopathy with idiopathic hyperammonaemia and Alzheimer type II astrocytes in equidae. Equine Vet J 1999;31:478–82.
12. Kitamura SS, Antonelli AC, Maruta CA, et al. A model for ammonia poisoning in cattle. Vet Hum Toxicol 2003;45:274–7.
13. Fernandez JM, Croom WJ Jr, Johnson AD, et al. Subclinical ammonia toxicity in steers: effects on blood metabolite and regulatory hormone concentrations. J Anim Sci 1988;66:3259–66.
14. McCornico RS, Duckett WM, Wood PA. Persistent hyperammonemia in two related Morgan weanlings. J Vet Intern Med 1997;11:264–6.
15. Bismuth M, Funakoshi N, Cadranel JF, et al. Hepatic encephalopathy: from pathophysiology to therapeutic management. Eur J Gastroenterol Hepatol 2011;23:8–22.
16. Fortier LA, Fubini SL, Flanders JA, et al. The diagnosis and surgical correction of congenital portosystemic vascular anomalies in two calves and two foals. Vet Surg 1996;25:154–60.
17. Lee JW. Fluid and electrolyte disturbances in critically ill patients. Electrolyte Blood Press 2010;8:72–81.
18. Passeron A, Dupeux S, Blanchard A. Hyponatremia: from physiopathology to practice. Rev Med Intern 2010;31:277–86.
19. Lakrtiz J, Madigan J, Carlson GP. Hypovolemic hyponatremia and signs of neurologic disease associated with diarrhea in a foal. J Am Vet Med Assoc 1992;200:1114–6.
20. Mortiz ML, Ayus JC. New aspects in the pathogenesis, prevention, and treatment of hyponatremic encephalopathy in children. Pediatr Nephrol 2010;25:1225–38.
21. Vaidya C, Ho W, Freda BJ. Management of hyponatremia: providing treatment and avoiding harm. Cleve Clin J Med 2010;77:715–26.
22. Hollis AR, Boston RC, Corley KTT. Plasma aldosterone, vasopressin and atrial natriuretic peptide in hypovolaemia: a preliminary comparative study of neonatal and mature horses. Equine Vet J 2008;40:64–9.

23. Pringle JK, Berthiaume LM. Hypernatremia in calves. J Vet Intern Med 1988;2:66–70.

24. Angelos SM, Smith BP, George LW, et al. Treatment of hypernatremia in an acidotic neonatal calf. J Am Vet Med Assoc 1999;214:1364–7.

25. Fang C, Mao J, Dai Y, et al. Fluid management of hypernatraemic dehydration to prevent cerebral oedema: a retrospective case control study of 97 children in China. J Paediatr Child Health 2010;46:301–3.

26. Loynachan AT, Williams NM, Freestone JF. Kernicterus in a neonatal foal. J Vet Diagn Invest 2007;19:209–12.

27. Hollis AR, Furr MO, Magdesian KG, et al. Blood glucose concentrations in critically ill neonatal foals. J Vet Intern Med 2008;22:1223–7.

28. Amaral AI, Teixeira AP, Sonnewald U, et al. Estimation of intracellular fluxes in cerebellar neurons after hypoglycemia: importance of the pyruvate recycling pathway and glutamine oxidation. J Neurosci Res 2011;89:700–10.

29. Lee BW, Jin ES, Hwang HS, et al. A case of hypoglycemic brain injuries with cortical laminar necrosis. J Korean Med Sci 2010;25:961–5.

30. Jain A, Aggarwal R, Sankar MJ. Hypoglycemia in the newborn. Indian J Pediatr 2010;77:1137–42.

31. Van den Berghe G, Wouters P, Weekers F, et al. Intensive insulin therapy in the critically ill patients. N Engl J Vet Med 2001;345:1359–67.

32. Chieregato A. Permissive mild to moderate hyperglycemia is safer for damaged brains. Minerva Anestesiol 2010;76:879–81.

33. Nadeem M, Murray DM, Boylan GB, et al. Early blood glucose profile and neurodevelopmental outcome at two years in neonatal hypoxic ischaemic encephalopathy. BMC Pediatr 2011;11:10.

34. Iwata O, Iwata S. Filling the evidence gap: how can we improve the outcome of neonatal encephalopathy in the next 10 years? Brain Dev 2010;33:221–8.

35. Wilcox AL, Calise DV, Chapman SE, et al. Hypoxic/ischemic encephalopathy associated with placental insufficiency in a cloned foal. Vet Pathol 2009;46:75–9.

36. Beyer MJ, Freestone JF, Reimer JM, et al. Idiopathic hypocalcemia in foals. J Vet Intern Med 1997;11:356–60.

37. Jain A, Agarwal R, Sankar MJ, et al. Hypocalcemia in the newborn. Indian J Pediatr 2010;77:1123–8.

Index

Note: Page numbers of article titles are in **boldface** type.

A

Acroptilon repens
  neurologic dysfunction in horses due to, 515, 521
Air embolus
  venous
    neurologic dysfunction in horses due to, 509–510
Anaplasma phagocytophilum infection
  equine nervous system effects of, 578
Anaplasmosis
  recumbency in adult horse due to, 536
Astragalus spp.
  neurologic dysfunction in horses due to, 515
Ataxia
  defined, 441
Autonomic innervation
  eye and, 466–468

B

Bacterial diseases
  equine nervous system effects of, 578–579
Blindness
  after intracarotid injections, 476
  central
    causes of, 474–476
  postanesthetic, 475–476
  sudden
    causes of, 469–476
      chorioretinitis, 473
      compressive optic neuropathy, 471
      exudative optic neuropathy, 473–474
      head trauma, 470–471
      ischemic or blood loss optic neuropathy, 472
      optic neuritis, 472
      retinal detachment, 473
      toxic neuropathy, 472–473
Blink reflex
  in neuro-ophthalmologic examination, 457, 464
Blood loss optic neuropathy
  sudden blindness in horse due to, 472

Moving?

Make sure your subscription moves with you!

To notify us of your new address, find your **Clinics Account Number** (located on your mailing label above your name), and contact customer service at:

Email: journalscustomerservice-usa@elsevier.com

800-654-2452 (subscribers in the U.S. & Canada)
314-447-8871 (subscribers outside of the U.S. & Canada)

Fax number: 314-447-8029

Elsevier Health Sciences Division
Subscription Customer Service
3251 Riverport Lane
Maryland Heights, MO 63043

*To ensure uninterrupted delivery of your subscription, please notify us at least 4 weeks in advance of move.

Printed and bound by CPI Group (UK) Ltd, Croydon, CR0 4YY

14/10/2024

01773668-0003